About the Authors

DR CAROLYN CHARMAN is a Consultant Dermatologist at the Royal Devon and Exeter Hospital. She trained as a Specialist Registrar in Dermatology at the Queen's Medical Centre – one of the UK's leading research centres, based at the University of Nottingham – where she developed a research interest in atopic eczema. She has a special interest in the causes and treatment of eczema, and has contributed to four recent books and several national and international publications on eczema and its management.

SANDRA LAWTON is Nurse Consultant Dermatology, Queen's Medical Centre, Nottingham. She has worked in dermatology for 19 years and developed the first dermatology liaison sister post in 1990. Her areas of interest include paediatric dermatology, care of children and their families with atopic eczema, nurse-led services in primary care and teledermatology.

D1510397

Acknowledgements

We would like to thank Jane Davison (Paediatric Dietician) and Dr David Thomas (Consultant Paediatrician) at the Queen's Medical Centre in Nottingham for their specialist advice and guidance during the production of this book. We are also grateful to the team at the National Eczema Society and to the Nottingham Support Group for Carers of Children with Eczema (www.nottinghameczema.org.uk) for reading the final drafts of the book and providing useful comments.

ECZEMA
WHAT REALLY WORKS
Treatments and Therapies

Carolyn Charman
and
Sandra Lawton

ROBINSON
London

Constable & Robinson Ltd
3 The Lanchesters
162 Fulham Palace Road
London W6 9ER
www.constablerobinson.com

First published in the UK by Robinson,
an imprint of Constable & Robinson Ltd 2006

A copy of the British Library Cataloguing in Publication
Data is available from the British Library.

ISBN-13: 978-1-84529-071-9
ISBN-10: 1-84529-071-2

Printed and bound in the EU

1 3 5 7 9 10 8 6 4 2

Contents

Foreword   vii
Introduction   viii

1 What is eczema?   1
■ *What does eczema look like?* ■ *How does eczema damage the skin?* ■ *Different types of eczema*

2 Causes and prevention of eczema   20
■ *Genetic factors* ■ *Environmental factors* ■ *Dietary factors* ■ *Reduced exposure to infection* ■ *Gravity* ■ *Stress*

3 Eczema and infections   45
■ *Bacterial infections* ■ *Viral infections* ■ *Fungal and yeast infections*

4 General advice on treating eczema   56
■ *Sources of help* ■ *Basic rules for treating eczema*

5 Emollients   62
■ *Choosing an emollient* ■ *How to use emollients* ■ *Common questions about emollients* ■ *Using emollients in different types of eczema*

6 Topical steroids   70
■ *Topical steroid strengths* ■ *Understanding topical steroids* ■ *How to use your topical steroids* ■ *Getting to grips with using different strengths of topical steroids*

7 Topical immunomodulators   92
■ *How to use topical immunomodulators* ■ *Using topical immunomodulators in different types of eczema*

8 **Bandages** 100
■ *Wet wrap bandaging* ■ *Dry wrapping* ■ *Medicated bandages*
■ *Compression bandages*

9 **Light therapy and tablet treatment** 107
■ *Light therapy* ■ *Tablet treatment*

10 **Alternative treatments and interventions** 118
■ *Complementary therapies* ■ *Psychological approaches*
■ *Dietary interventions* ■ *Salt baths*

11 **Allergy tests and eczema** 132
■ *What is an allergy?* ■ *The role of allergy in eczema*
■ *Allergy tests in eczema*

12 **Nursery and school** 155
■ *Nursery and playgroup* ■ *School*

13 **Social life and leisure** 168
■ *Sports* ■ *Holidays* ■ *Growing up*

14 **The impact of eczema on feelings, emotions and
relationships** 178
■ *Tiredness and exhaustion* ■ *Guilt and depression*
■ *Anxiety and worry* ■ *Irritability* ■ *Relationships* ■ *Summary*

Glossary 195
Resources 198
Index 205

Foreword

I have always found it rather strange that so little attention has been paid to eczema in the UK. Atopic eczema now affects around 20 per cent of all British school children, and other forms of eczema are among the most common reasons for seeing a family doctor about a skin problem, yet the quality and quantity of good advice to the public are sadly lacking. This book, by Dr Carolyn Charman and Nurse Consultant Sandra Lawton, goes a long way to redressing that balance. This book is not only for people with eczema, but also for those who live with, and care for, eczema sufferers. It is a *practical* guide, written in a helpful question-and-answer format – questions that are not made up for the sake of writing the book, but ones that have been generated during years of experience in working *with* eczema sufferers and their families at the award-winning special eczema clinic at the Queen's Medical Centre, Nottingham. Unlike some dubious sources of printed and electronic eczema advice that I have come across in the past, Charman and Lawton strive to base their answers on good quality and up-to-date external research evidence where this is available. It is hoped that this will help to dispel some of the myths and rituals surrounding eczema that you might have been bullied into believing in the past. Although there is still much we do not know about eczema, this book will help you understand more about what we do know in an explicit, positive and practical way.

Professor Hywel Williams
Director of the Centre of Evidence-Based Dermatology at
the University of Nottingham, UK

Introduction

Welcome to *Eczema*. If you suffer from eczema or look after children with the condition, this book is for you. It is designed to take you through everything you need to know about eczema, from causes and prevention to effective treatment, in a simple step-by-step fashion. The book gives practical explanations for all the commonly asked questions, ranging from daily skin care to the latest advances in treatment and research. It is full of useful tips designed to help you tailor treatment to your own individual lifestyle. By giving you a deeper understanding of your own skin this book will help you stay in control of your eczema in the safest and most effective way possible. If you are a parent of a child with eczema the information in this book can be applied to the care of your child in exactly the same way as if you are an eczema sufferer yourself. Although the book cannot substitute for individual advice from your own doctor or nurse, it will help you get lots more out of your consultations with healthcare professionals, and allow you to use all the help that is available to maximum benefit. So read on to discover just what we mean by eczema, and how to recognize it.

Chapter 1
What is eczema?

Eczema is a common skin condition which can affect anyone at any age – from early infancy to old age. Another name for eczema is dermatitis (from *derma*, meaning skin, and *-itis*, meaning inflammation). Skin inflammation is the main feature of eczema. This inflammation is caused by cells and chemicals in your immune system. The cells and chemicals react inside the skin in a complicated way and cause skin damage. The inflammation irritates the nerve endings in this skin and this makes you feel very itchy.

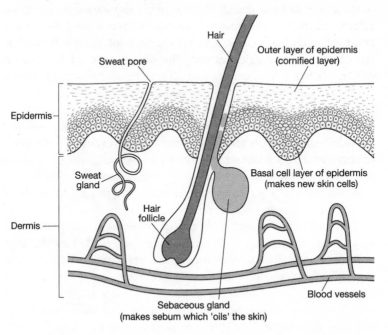

Cross-section of the skin.

What does eczema look like?

Eczema changes the appearance of the skin. In mild eczema the skin may just be a bit pink and scaly. If there is more inflammation the skin becomes red and bumpy, and may blister or weep clear liquid (the word 'eczema' actually comes from the Greek for 'boiling', which describes the tiny blisters or bubbles that are often seen in early eczema). In dark-skinned people the patches of eczema may look dark rather than red. Sometimes, yellow crusts, scabs or pus-filled spots appear on the skin, especially if the eczema becomes infected. In longstanding eczema the skin can become thickened, leathery and cracked, especially on the hands and feet or around the joints. Constant scratching and inflammation can leave dark or pale patches on the skin – they eventually return to normal when the eczema is controlled. These colour changes occur in all skin types, but the darker a person's skin is to start with, the more obvious they look. The exact combination of skin changes varies a lot from person to person so that no two people will find that their eczema is identical. Although eczema may look unpleasant, it is not infectious so you cannot catch it from someone who has it or pass it on.

How does eczema damage the skin?

Your skin forms an important barrier between you and the outside world, and is therefore crucial in preventing you from losing too much water or heat from your body, and in keeping germs out. Your skin is made up of a thin outer layer called the *epidermis* and a thicker layer underneath called the *dermis*. Both of these layers contain cells, water, fats and oils.

The smoothness and softness of your skin depends on a balance of water, fats and oils in your epidermis. Healthy skin cells contain lots of water. In people with eczema the skin produces less fats and oils. Without a good 'mortar', the skin cells dry out and shrink, leaving gaps in the skin barrier through which more water can be lost. These gaps also allow germs and harmful substances from the environment to get into the skin more easily. Although these gaps may initially be too small to see, they soon become visible as cracks and fissures if the eczema continues.

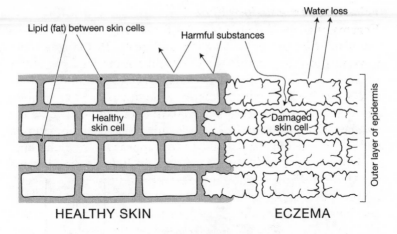

The outer layer of the epidermis is like a strong brick wall which keeps moisture in the skin and harmful substances out. The skin cells produce lipid (a fatty substance) which acts like mortar, holding the cells (bricks) together. Healthy skin cells are plump with water and fit tightly together to form a strong barrier. In eczema the mortar is not formed properly, allowing the skin cells to dry out and leave gaps in the wall. Once the skin barrier is damaged harmful substances (allergens and irritants) can get into the skin and cause further inflammation and damage.

Different types of eczema

There are different types of eczema, based on the appearance, distribution and cause. It is important to know which type of eczema you have because some types of eczema tend to last much longer than others, and the causes are not the same for each type. Your doctor will usually be able to tell you which type of eczema you have by listening to your symptoms and examining your skin. The most common types of eczema are:

- atopic eczema
- seborrhoeic eczema
- contact eczema
- discoid eczema
- pompholyx eczema
- asteatotic eczema
- gravitational eczema.

Atopic eczema

Atopic eczema, also called atopic dermatitis, is the most common form of eczema, especially in children. The condition now affects

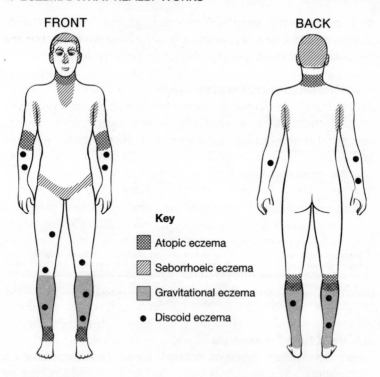

FRONT

BACK

Key

▨ Atopic eczema

▧ Seborrhoeic eczema

▦ Gravitational eczema

● Discoid eczema

Common sites on the body to be affected by different types of eczema.

up to a fifth of school children in the UK, and in some of these children it continues into adulthood. The number of people suffering from atopic eczema has more than doubled over the last thirty to forty years, although the reasons for this are still not completely clear. 'Atopic' is a term used to describe a tendency to develop eczema, asthma or hayfever. In all of these conditions the body's immune system overreacts to common things in the environment that would normally not cause any harm. These common things include pollen, animal fur, foods and house dust mites. Atopic eczema, asthma and hayfever often occur together in individuals or in families. In any individual atopic eczema usually develops first, followed by asthma and then hayfever at a later age. It is also common for people with atopic eczema to have other family members affected by atopic eczema, asthma or hayfever. It is impossible to predict exactly who will develop these other atopic diseases. This means that if you have atopic eczema you will not necessarily get asthma or hayfever, but the risk is higher than for people without atopic eczema.

Q. How is atopic eczema diagnosed?

Atopic eczema is diagnosed by its appearance and symptoms. It usually affects the skin creases (flexures) around the elbows, knees and ankles but can involve any part of the body. In babies and young infants it often develops on the face and scalp first, and the nappy area is often unaffected. As with other types of eczema the skin becomes red and inflamed, and may ooze or weep or just look dry and scaly. Atopic eczema is very itchy and children may scratch through the day and night. Young babies with atopic eczema often rub their faces on their sheets or clothes.

Although the symptoms and signs of atopic eczema are usually characteristic it can sometimes be difficult to diagnose the condition, especially in children under the age of one. A simple guide for you and your doctor is given below. This can be used to help diagnose atopic eczema in adults or children.

Atopic eczema is diagnosed when you have an itchy rash or are repeatedly scratching or rubbing your skin, and have three or more of the following symptoms:

- the itchy rash is present in skin creases such as the folds of the elbows, behind the knees, in front of the ankles or around the neck (or the cheeks in children less than four years old)
- a history of asthma or hayfever (or a history of asthma, eczema or hayfever in an immediate relative, in children less than four years old)
- generally dry skin in the past year
- visible eczema in the skin creases (or eczema affecting the cheeks, forehead, or outer part of the arms or legs in children less than four years old) – ask your doctor to confirm the presence of visible eczema if you are unsure
- onset of the itchy rash in the first two years of life.

These criteria were developed by the UK Atopic Dermatitis Diagnostic Criteria Working Party.

Q. Can blood tests be used to diagnose atopic eczema?

No. There are no blood tests that can tell you whether you definitely have atopic eczema or not. People with atopic eczema often have high levels in their blood of an antibody called immunoglobulin E (IgE). Antibodies are proteins that form part of the body's immune system. Around 80 per cent of people with atopic eczema have high levels of IgE. However, the levels of IgE vary a lot between different people and do not always reflect the severity of the eczema. Furthermore, many people with atopic eczema have normal IgE levels, so the test is not very accurate. As yet no other chemicals or proteins in the blood have been shown to be clearly linked with atopic eczema, and therefore the diagnosis is usually based on the combination of signs and symptoms discussed above.

Q. Who can get atopic eczema?

Atopic eczema is more common in children than in adults. It affects around a fifth of children in Western Europe, but becomes gradually less common with increasing age. In fact only 2 per cent of people aged between 16 and 40 years are affected, and less than 0.2 per cent of adults over the age of 40 years. Around 70 per cent of children who have atopic eczema develop it in the first five years of life, and 60 to 70 per cent of affected children will be free of the disease by their early teenage years.

Q. Does atopic eczema run in families?

Yes, as mentioned above, it often does, but not always. Atopic eczema, asthma and hayfever are all related and often run in families. However, the way in which these atopic conditions is inherited varies. Atopic eczema is not always passed directly from parent to child, but the risk of a child developing eczema increases if family members are affected, as shown below.

- If a child has no parents, brothers or sisters with eczema, asthma or hayfever his or her risk of developing atopic eczema is around 1:10 (10 per cent).
- If a child has one parent with eczema, asthma or hayfever then the risk of the child developing atopic eczema is around 1:4 (25 per cent).

- If a child has a brother or sister with eczema, asthma or hayfever then the risk of his or her developing atopic eczema is between 1:4 and 1:2 (25 to 50 per cent).
- If both of a child's parents have eczema, asthma or hayfever then the risk of the child developing atopic eczema is around 1:2 (50 per cent).

Q. Are boys more likely than girls to get atopic eczema?

No, little evidence exists that there is any real difference in risk between boys and girls. Some studies have found that in children of school age atopic eczema is slightly more common in girls, although in very young infants other studies have found that a few more boys are affected. However, overall no big difference has been demonstrated.

Q. Is atopic eczema more common among black children than white children?

In the UK the frequency of atopic eczema appears to be similar in white children compared with Asian children. However, atopic eczema is almost twice as common in Afro-Caribbean children born in the UK compared with white children. In other parts of the world similar differences are seen between different ethnic groups. For example, Chinese children born in the USA or Australia are much more likely to develop eczema that local white children.

Q. Is atopic eczema more common in big rather than small families?

Plenty of research has found that atopic eczema is more common in children from smaller families. Unlike many other diseases atopic eczema is also more common in families with higher incomes.

Q. Does the frequency of atopic eczema vary across the world?

Yes, it does. Interestingly, just as atopic eczema is more common in families with higher incomes, the disease is also much more common in wealthy countries compared with less-developed parts of the world. Some of the highest rates of eczema are seen in Northern and Western Europe and other countries with a

Westernized lifestyle and market economy. Much lower rates are seen in China, Central Asia and Eastern Europe. An ongoing worldwide study called the International Study of Asthma and Allergies in Childhood is investigating and monitoring these worldwide differences in the rates of atopic eczema to help identify important causes.

Q. Does the frequency of atopic eczema vary across the UK?
Yes, it does. Research studies have shown that atopic eczema is more common in southern and eastern areas of the country, although the exact reasons remain unclear.

Q. Will I grow out of my atopic eczema?
On an individual basis it is impossible to predict who will grow out of their eczema, although overall around three-quarters of people will be clear of the condition by adulthood. Atopic eczema is more likely to continue into adulthood if you have severe widespread eczema starting very early in life, asthma or hayfever as well, and other family members with eczema. There is no proof that any of the treatments used for atopic eczema have any effect on how long it takes for a person to grow out of the disease.

Seborrhoeic eczema

Seborrhoeic eczema, also called seborrhoeic dermatitis, is a very common and usually mild type of eczema which affects both very young children and adults. 'Seborrhoeic' means greasy or oily – this type of eczema affects areas of skin where natural grease (sebum) production is high. Although it is still not absolutely clear why people develop seborrhoeic eczema, it is known that common yeasts that live on the skin may be significant. These yeasts like areas of skin where there are lots of grease glands, such as the face and scalp, and are discussed in more detail in Chapter 2.

In children seborrhoeic eczema develops in the first few months of life and usually affects the scalp and skin creases. Thick, yellow, greasy scales and crusts are seen on the scalp (the condition is often called cradle cap). Scales may also develop around the nose, forehead, eyebrows and behind the ears. The nappy area and armpits are often affected too. The skin may look inflamed, red and glistening. Sometimes oozing and crusting develop too. Seborrhoeic eczema can spread to involve other areas of skin, giving blotchy red scaly patches which merge into each other. Fortunately the condition is not usually itchy and often doesn't bother the child at all, although it may look unpleasant.

In adults seborrhoeic eczema is more common in men than women, but can affect both genders. It is most common in young to middle-aged adults and usually starts as dandruff on the scalp, which may spread to the face and neck. The forehead, ears, eyebrows, eyelids and folds at the side of the nose are most often affected. The skin looks yellowish-red with small white flakes of skin and sometimes crusts. Patches of seborrhoeic eczema may also develop on the centre of the chest or back, in the armpits and groins or under the breasts. In adults the condition is much less itchy than atopic eczema, but it can be irritating and cosmetically troublesome.

Q. Does seborrhoeic eczema run in families?

No, unlike atopic eczema there is no evidence that seborrhoeic eczema runs in families.

Q. How long does seborrhoeic eczema last for?

The majority of young babies grow out of their seborrhoeic eczema between the ages of six and twelve months. Adult seborrhoeic eczema can last for months or years, although it becomes gradually less common with increasing age.

Contact dermatitis

Contact dermatitis, also called contact eczema, is a type of eczema caused by substances coming into contact with the skin. Many different substances can cause contact dermatitis, including common things in the home or work environment. Contact dermatitis can be divided into two types: irritant contact dermatitis and allergic contact dermatitis.

Irritant contact dermatitis is very common, accounting for over three-quarters of cases of contact dermatitis. It occurs as a direct result of physical damage to the skin by substances such as soaps, detergents, solvents and diluted acids or alkalis. These substances irritate the skin without a person actually becoming allergic to them, and the more contact one has with the substance the more irritated one's skin becomes. Irritant contact dermatitis is most commonly seen on the hands, especially around the finger webs, where the skin is delicate and prone to damage. Occasionally the fingernails can become thickened and dented if the problem affects the hands for any length of time. The skin changes range from mild dryness to severe redness, cracking and blistering.

Allergic contact dermatitis is much less common than irritant contact dermatitis, accounting for around a fifth of cases of contact dermatitis overall. It occurs when a person becomes allergic to something coming into contact with the skin (see Chapter 11). This means that your body's immune system starts reacting against that substance and remembers it, so that every time you come into contact with it again you develop eczema. Once you have developed a contact allergy, even small amounts of contact with the substance will cause eczema. Allergic contact dermatitis is often seen on the hands but can affect any area of skin. If the skin around the nails is affected then the nails can become abnormal and thickened. The distribution of the eczema often gives a clue to the cause as it usually occurs only where the substance has been in contact with the skin. Occasionally contact dermatitis can spread to other parts of the body that haven't been in direct contact with the substance. The skin changes can range from mild redness and scaling to severe inflammation with weeping, cracking and blistering. The affected skin is usually very itchy and sore.

Q. How can I tell the difference between irritant and allergic contact dermatitis?

Although the history and distribution of the skin changes can give a clue, irritant and allergic contact dermatitis can often look very similar. A special form of allergy test is sometimes needed to tell the difference and confirm what substances are causing the problem. These allergy tests are called patch tests, and they are described in detail in Chapter 11. Patch tests are positive if you have an allergic contact dermatitis and negative if you have an irritant contact dermatitis.

Q. Who can get irritant contact dermatitis?

Irritant contact dermatitis can affect anyone of any age. It is the most common cause of occupational-related skin disease, and particularly tends to affect people in occupations involving wet work, such as catering, hairdressing, cleaning, nursing and cooking. It is a common cause of hand eczema in women looking after the home, especially if they are also caring for young children. People with a history of atopy (atopic eczema, hayfever or asthma) are more prone to getting irritant contact dermatitis as their skin is more sensitive and vulnerable to damage.

Q. Who can get allergic contact dermatitis?

Anyone, both young and old, can get allergic contact dermatitis. Research suggests that the risk of allergic contact dermatitis is not higher in people with atopic eczema, in contrast to irritant contact dermatitis. Allergic contact dermatitis usually develops in people who are regularly exposed to particular substances. For example, women and girls are at increased risk of developing allergic contact dermatitis to nickel because this is found in earrings and metal jewellery. People with leg ulcers are particularly likely to develop allergic contact dermatitis to creams and ointments or rubber in their bandages. Keen gardeners or florists are at risk of developing allergic contact dermatitis to plants such as chrysanthemums and alstroemeria. Bricklayers may develop contact allergy to chromate, a substance found in cement. The list of possible causes is endless. People often think that they cannot become allergic to something they have been using for a long time but this isn't true. Allergic contact dermatitis can develop after months or years of exposure with no previous problems.

Q. What are the most common causes of contact allergic dermatitis?

The most common things to cause allergic contact dermatitis include nickel (in some jewellery), fragrances (in perfumes and toiletries), preservatives (in creams and ointments), antibiotic creams, hair dyes, rubber (in gloves, balloons, condoms), chromate (in leather and cement) and plants.

Q. How long does contact dermatitis tend to last?

Irritant contact dermatitis will usually clear up quickly if you can modify your lifestyle and avoid the irritant substances as much as possible. Similarly, most types of allergic contact dermatitis will clear if the substance causing the problem can be identified and avoided. Some causes of allergic contact dermatitis are easier to avoid than others. For instance, it is relatively easy to avoid hair dyes or rubber gloves but it may be much more difficult to completely avoid fragrances, which can be carried in the air from perfumes or air-fresheners. Contact allergic dermatitis caused by plants can also cause intermittent symptoms for years, especially in the summer, when plant material can be carried around in the air and cause problems on exposed sites such as the face. A few substances can cause contact allergic dermatitis that can carry on for years even when the substance is completely avoided – an example is chromate in cement. Very occasionally contact allergic dermatitis can make the skin more sensitive to sunlight and this can cause ongoing skin inflammation in the spring and summer months, even when the substance is avoided.

Discoid eczema

Discoid eczema, also called nummular eczema, is a less common type of eczema which develops as round coin-shaped patches of scaly skin about the size of a fifty-pence piece or smaller. They can occur anywhere on the body but most often affect the lower legs or arms. The skin is itchy, red and bumpy, and can become very inflamed, with oozing and crusting, especially if the eczema becomes infected. As the eczema clears the patches become dry and scaly.

Q. Who can get discoid eczema?

Anyone can get discoid eczema although it is most common in older children and adults who have very dry skin. It does not usually run in families, and is not usually associated with asthma or hayfever.

Q. Can discoid and atopic eczema occur together?

The term discoid eczema is usually used when coin-shaped patches of eczema occur as the only manifestation of eczema.

However, some people with atopic eczema do develop round stubborn patches of eczema along with the more typical eczema in the skin creases.

Q. How long does discoid eczema last?

This is very variable. The patches will clear with treatment, but over time the same patches of eczema can flare up again and again, or new patches can develop. This can continue for months or sometimes even years.

Pompholyx eczema

Pompholyx eczema, also called dyshidrotic eczema, is a blistering type of eczema which affects the hands and feet. 'Pompholyx' means blisters, and 'dyshidrotic' means altered sweating. This type of eczema was originally thought to be related to sweating, but no clear link has ever been proven. Often, no primary cause for the eczema is found. Pompholyx eczema often appears quite suddenly. Some people notice a warm or prickling sensation before the eczema develops. Crops of blisters containing clear fluid then appear on the hands, feet or both. The size of the blisters can range from very tiny (a few millimetres) to big (a few centimetres). Tiny blisters often occur along the sides of the fingers, whereas bigger blisters affect other parts of the hands or feet where the skin is much thicker. Blisters on the palms and soles can be very deep-seated – they can look a bit like tapioca. The blisters are extremely itchy, and as they clear up the skin can become very scaly, red and cracked.

Q. Who can get pompholyx eczema?

It is most common in young adults and doesn't occur very often in children under ten years or adults over 40 years.

Q. Are the hands affected more often than the feet?

Yes. In around eight out of ten people only the hands are affected. The feet are affected in around one in ten people, and both the hands and the feet also in one in ten people. Pompholyx eczema accounts for less than a fifth of cases of hand eczema, so it is much less common than contact dermatitis or atopic eczema.

Q. How long do the blisters last?

Usually the blisters clear up over two or three weeks, but they may come back again after a few weeks or months. Overall, pompholyx eczema can continue off and on for several months or even years.

Asteatotic eczema

Asteatotic eczema, also called eczema craquelé or winter eczema, is a type of eczema associated with very dry skin. It most often affects the shins, but sometimes involves other areas such as the thighs, arms, stomach and back. The skin becomes rough and scaly. Affected areas may show a criss-cross pattern of cracks that look like 'crazy-paving' or 'a dried river bed.' The cracks affect only the very top layers of the skin but can look very red and feel sore or itchy. It is uncommon to see blistering or thickening of the skin in this type of eczema.

Q. Who can get asteatotic eczema?

Asteatotic eczema occurs most commonly in people over the age of 60. This is because skin becomes drier as you get older. Elderly people living in dry heated rooms or those exposed to winter weather or excessive bathing or showering are all at risk of developing this type of eczema.

Q. How long does asteatotic eczema last?

Untreated, this type of eczema can last for weeks or months but it usually responds to simple lifestyle changes and mild treatments (see Chapters 2 and 5).

Gravitational eczema

Gravitational eczema, also called stasis eczema or varicose eczema, is a common type of eczema related to increased pressure in the veins of the legs. Blood travels down the legs in vessels called arteries, and is pumped back up to the heart through vessels called veins. Over time in some people leg veins become less good at returning blood to the heart. The blood then pools up in the legs, and the increased pressure forces fluid out of the veins and into the skin. Gradually this makes the skin of the lower legs become shiny, red, itchy and flaky. This is called gravitational eczema. Small speckled red-brown spots of leaked blood can appear in the skin, especially around the inside of the ankle. You may also get some ankle swelling. Sometimes the eczema can become weepy and oozy, and over a period of time the skin can become very thickened and leathery.

Q. Who can get gravitational eczema?

Gravitational eczema is most common in adults who have varicose veins or who have a history of leg ulcers or blood clots (deep vein thrombosis) in the legs. However, some people develop increased pressure in their leg veins without ever having had varicose veins, leg ulcers or blood clots. Other risk factors include being overweight or spending a lot of time standing up. Gravitational eczema is more common in women than men because female hormones and pregnancy both increase the risk of developing the condition.

Q. How long does gravitational eczema last?

Gravitational eczema can be an ongoing problem for many people because the increased pressure in their leg veins persist and often gets worse with time. The problem can be kept under control and the risk of it progressing can be reduced by using the treatments discussed in Chapters 5 and 6, and the regular use of compression stockings to support the legs (Chapter 8). A few people can reduce the pressure in their leg veins by losing weight or undergoing surgery to their leg veins.

Q. Can gravitational eczema affect other areas of the body?

Usually gravitational eczema is restricted to the lower legs because this is where the pressure of blood in the veins is highest (because humans walk upright). However, occasionally the eczema can spread to involve the whole of the legs or even cause a widespread eczema. This is most likely to occur if your gravitational eczema is severe and not being controlled with proper treatment.

Q. Is gravitational eczema related to leg ulcers?

Yes, but having gravitational eczema does not mean that you will necessarily develop a leg ulcer. Increased pressure in the leg veins is one of the most common causes of leg ulcers, and people with gravitational eczema are at an increased risk of developing leg ulcers, particularly in the damaged areas of skin. Ulcers usually start after minor trauma such as scratching the eczema or banging your leg, so extra care is needed. Leg ulcers can be very slow to heal because of the sluggish blood flow to and from the skin. Sometimes a leg ulcer will develop before the gravitational eczema appears. Usually the eczema develops as patches of itchy red flaky skin around the edge of the ulcer. It is important to remember that allergic contact dermatitis is another possible cause of lower leg eczema in people with leg ulcers, and it can look similar to gravitational eczema. The contact allergy is usually caused by the creams, dressings or bandages that are being used to treat the ulcer. Sometimes allergic contact dermatitis and gravitational eczema occur together. Your doctor will arrange patch testing to exclude a contact allergy if necessary.

Other skin conditions that can be mistaken for eczema

There are lots of different skin conditions that can look like eczema. The common ones are discussed below. If you are in any doubt your GP or local dermatologist will help make a correct diagnosis.

Psoriasis

Psoriasis can be mistaken for atopic, discoid or seborrhoeic eczema. It is a very common inflammatory skin condition which affects around 1 in 100 people.

Q. What does psoriasis look like?

Psoriasis develops as pink patches of skin covered by silvery white scale. It can affect any part of the body, although by far the most common sites are the knees and elbows. The scalp is often affected, giving bad dandruff and thick scaling. The nails can become thickened and may develop small dents (pits) in them.

Q. How can I tell the difference between psoriasis and eczema?

Psoriasis usually affects the front of the knees and bony parts of the elbows. In contrast, atopic eczema usually affects the skin creases behind the knees or inside the elbows. Another clue is the amount of itching. Psoriasis may be slightly itchy but is not usually anywhere near as itchy as eczema. People with psoriasis may have other family members affected by psoriasis whereas people with atopic eczema are more likely to have family members with eczema, asthma or hayfever. On the scalp it can be very difficult to tell the difference between psoriasis and seborrhoeic eczema unless other parts of the body are affected too.

Ringworm

Ringworm (sometimes called tinea) can sometimes be mistaken for eczema. Ringworm is a common skin infection caused by a fungus (called a dermatophyte) which spreads in the top layers of the skin. There are many different types of ringworm fungus. Some are spread from person to person while others are picked up from the soil, or from animals like cats, dogs or cattle.

Q. What does ringworm look like?

On the feet: The most common type of ringworm is athlete's foot, which is especially common in people who do lots of sport. The fungus is often picked up in swimming pools and loves hot sweaty feet (for example, in trainers). Athlete's foot appears as itchy scaly patches between the toes which may spread onto the foot or cause thickening and discolouration of the toenails. Very occasionally ringworm on the feet results in a blistering eczema on the palms of the hands which looks like pompholyx eczema – this is called an 'id' reaction.

On the body: The ringworm fungus can affect any part of the body. If the feet are affected the ringworm may spread to the groins to give itchy red patches that gradually spread down the thighs. On the body ringworm causes circular red patches with scaling around the edge. The skin in the middle of the patch often clears up as the patch expands outwards.

On the scalp: Scalp ringworm mainly affects children and produces itching, scaling and patches of broken hair or hair loss.

Q. How can I tell the difference between ringworm and eczema?

Athlete's foot is usually easy to recognize, but round patches of ringworm on the body can look very like eczema, especially discoid eczema. Scalp eczema very rarely causes hair loss, so if you develop patches of hair loss with scaling see your doctor to exclude ringworm. The ringworm fungus is easily detected in skin scale and hair samples which your doctor can send off to the laboratory if necessary. If ringworm is mistakenly treated as eczema with steroid creams it will continue to spread and may alter its appearance so it becomes more difficult to diagnose.

Nappy rash

Nappy rash, sometimes called napkin dermatitis, can sometimes be mistaken for childhood seborrhoeic eczema or atopic eczema. It is caused by irritation from urine coming into contact with the skin. It is more likely to occur if nappies are not changed frequently, although some babies are just very prone to developing the problem even with regular changes. It can usually be prevented by using barrier creams with every nappy change.

Q. What does nappy rash look like?

Nappy rash develops as red patches of skin around the baby's genital area. Sometimes the skin becomes weepy and scaly. Thrush (*candida*) is a common yeast infection which can infect nappy rash, causing tiny white pus-filled spots on the skin. If this occurs your doctor can prescribe an anti-thrush cream.

Q. How can I tell the difference between nappy rash and eczema?

Nappy rash doesn't affect other areas of the body, and often spares the skin creases in the groins because they are not in close contact with the nappy. This is the opposite of seborrhoeic eczema, which tends to affect the skin creases. Nappy rash is usually sore rather than itchy, so scratching is less common than in babies with eczema.

Scabies

Scabies is a very itchy skin condition caused by infection by an eight-legged mite. It is spread by close contact with an infected person, and can affect anyone from small children to the elderly. It can spread very rapidly where lots of people are close together, such as in nursing homes or schools. The mite burrows into the top layers of the skin to lay eggs. Usually only ten or so mites infect the skin but this is enough to cause symptoms. The itching occurs because your body's immune system reacts against the mite and its droppings. The itching takes four to six weeks to develop after a first infection, but if you have had scabies before the symptoms can start after only a few days. The itching associated with scabies is very intense and widespread, but doesn't usually affect the head and neck in adults.

Q. What does scabies look like?
There may be very little to see on the skin except scratch marks. Tiny ridges or tracks (less than 1cm long) can sometimes be seen. These tracks are burrows caused by the mite tunnelling into the skin. Burrows are best seen between the fingers, under the arms or in the genital area. In children burrows often affect the feet and can cause blistering. Crusting, scaling and firm purple lumps or nodules (usually less than 1cm big) can develop in the skin over time.

Q. How can I tell the difference between scabies and eczema?
If other family members or friends become itchy around the same time, there is a good chance that you have a scabies infection. The typical redness and scaling of eczema is not usually seen, and the skin rash may not be very obvious. Remember that scabies can occur in anyone, including people who already have underlying eczema.

Chapter 2
Causes and prevention of eczema

'What causes eczema?' is one of the most common questions people ask about the condition, but unfortunately there is no simple answer. Eczema is a very complicated disease which is thought to be *multifactorial* in origin – this means that lots of different factors play a part in its development. The factors that are important in causing eczema in one person may not be exactly the same in another person. Furthermore, in any individual many different overlapping and interacting causes usually play a role. What this means in practice is that avoiding any one cause is very unlikely to prevent or cure the eczema by itself. Avoidance of the causes discussed in this chapter will certainly improve many people's eczema significantly. Despite this, very few people will find that their eczema clears up completely, and most will still need some form of treatment. This is because many of the factors known to play a role are difficult to avoid completely (such as house dust mites), and some simply cannot be changed (such as the genes you are born with). It is also likely that there are important causes that medical research has not yet identified, although research is advancing all the time, and it is hoped that over the coming years we will come to understand much more about this complicated disease.

This chapter takes you through the many different factors that are thought to be important in causing and triggering eczema. It gives you sensible guidance on how to avoid making your eczema worse, and presents an up-to-date understanding of the factors that are thought to be most important in disease development.

Genetic factors
The genes that you inherit from your father and mother when you are born certainly play an important role in causing atopic

eczema, although genetic factors are less clearly involved in other types of eczema. Genes are bits of information that are carried in every cell of the body on structures called chromosomes. We know that genes are relevant to eczema because atopic eczema often runs in families, although the inheritance pattern is not always clear-cut. You are much more likely to develop atopic eczema if your mother or father suffered from the condition, with an even greater risk if both your parents have had the condition. Atopic eczema is also much more common in identical twins, who share the same genetic information in their cells, compared with non-identical twins. The genes involved in atopic eczema development are probably also important in other atopic diseases such as asthma and hayfever, which often run along with atopic eczema. So far no single gene has been identified as being responsible for atopic eczema development, although many have been implicated as possible contributors. It seems likely that the pattern of genes you are born with affects how likely you are to develop atopic eczema when you are exposed to other causes and triggers in the environment, with genetic and environmental factors interacting in a very complex way which varies between individuals.

Q. Is it possible to alter the genes you are born with?

As yet it is not possible to change or manipulate the genes you are born with. Gene technology is increasingly being applied to a number of medical conditions, but mainly on an experimental basis. However, gene therapy research is advancing and may offer some hope for the future if the most important eczema genes can be pin-pointed.

Q. My husband had eczema as a child and we are now expecting our first baby. Will he or she develop eczema?

There is no definite way of predicting if your baby will have eczema. Because it is not yet known which genes are responsible for eczema and how they are passed on, it is difficult to give accurate figures on the risk of your baby getting eczema. However, research studies have suggested that if only one parent has atopic eczema, asthma or hayfever then there is around a 1:4 (25 per cent) chance that your baby could develop atopic eczema, compared with around a 1:10 (10 per cent) chance in the general population.

Environmental factors

The dramatic rise in atopic eczema over the last forty to fifty years is thought to be partly related to changes in the environment in which we live, both inside and outside the home. Interestingly, the highest rates of atopic eczema are seen in affluent countries associated with a modern comfortable lifestyle. Other types of eczema such as asteatotic eczema, discoid eczema, contact eczema and pompholyx eczema may also be aggravated by environmental factors. So what specific factors in the environment are thought to contribute to eczema development?

House dust mite

House dust mites are thought to play a role in causing atopic eczema although they have not been specifically linked to other types of eczema. They are also thought to play a role in asthma.

Q. Someone told me that house dust mites could make atopic eczema worse. The thought makes me feel dirty. What are they?

House dust mites are tiny insects that are invisible to the human eye. They live on dead human skin cells and are found worldwide. They live in bedding, carpets, soft furnishings and soft toys, and can be found in all houses, clean or dirty. House dust mites thrive best at temperatures of between 17°C and 24°C, especially in damp humid conditions. This means that they like centrally heated insulated houses, particularly when there is plenty of soft furnishing for them to live in. Modern well-insulated houses with central heating, wall-to-wall carpets and soft furnishings are much more common nowadays than a few decades ago, and seem to provide the ideal environment for house dust mites to proliferate.

Q. How do house dust mites cause eczema?

For most people house dust mites are absolutely harmless. However, up to 80 per cent of people with atopic eczema have raised levels of antibody (IgE) to house dust mites and their faecal droppings, indicating that their immune systems have become sensitized or allergic to the mite. This allergy can cause symptoms such as redness and itching when their skin comes into contact with house dust mite particles in the environment. House dust mites can possibly also irritate the skin directly, even in people with no raised mite IgE levels. House dust mites are most likely to cause eczema by coming into direct contact with the skin, but they can also be carried in the air and become inhaled into the lungs – this route of contact can worsen asthma and potentially also make eczema worse. Although many people with atopic eczema have raised IgE levels to house dust mite, one of the problems linking the mite directly with eczema has been that IgE antibody is usually associated with immediate-type allergy (see Chapter 11). In the skin immediate-type allergies usually produce a skin rash called urticaria (or hives) which looks like a nettle rash rather than eczema. Urticaria usually develops very quickly and fades over a few hours, unlike eczema. However, over recent years it has been increasingly recognized that raised IgE levels can also be associated with delayed-type allergic reactions which look much more like typical eczema (see Chapter 11). This occurs through complicated interactions between cells and chemicals in the skin.

Q. If I reduce the house dust mite levels in my home will it make my eczema better?

Over many years researchers have looked at the effect of avoidance measures of house dust mites in great depth. Several clinical trials have studied patients closely (often over several months) to work out how much avoidance of house dust mites (using the measures described below) actually does improve atopic eczema. Unfortunately the answer is still not clear as studies have shown conflicting results. Some studies have shown an overall improvement in the sample of patients studied, especially when very low house dust mite levels were obtained. However, several other studies have shown no significant overall benefit, even when a lot of time and effort is put into keeping mite levels down. People with positive allergy tests to house dust mites (see Chapter 11) are most likely to benefit, but even with allergy testing it is impossible to predict which individuals will improve and which won't. As house dust mites may not play a role in everybody's eczema current research is focusing on developing better tests (such as the atopy patch test – see Chapter 11) to predict who will benefit most from avoidance.

Q. What does this mean for me in practice?

Measures to keep house dust mite levels down can be time-consuming and sometimes costly. In practice if someone in your family suffers from atopic eczema it is sensible to follow first the simple measures described below, such as regular vacuuming and buying bedding covers that are impermeable to house dust mites. More extreme measures include replacing carpets with vinyl floors. However, as yet there is not enough evidence to recommend such measures to everyone with atopic eczema as part of their routine care. If the eczema is mild and can be controlled safely with simple treatments then extreme changes to your home may not be necessary. Also, remember that most children will grow out of their eczema during childhood.

Q. What are the best ways of getting rid of house dust mites?

It is not usually possible to get rid of all the house dust mites in your home completely, but you can keep the levels down by following these measures.

- Vacuum carpets and mattresses regularly with a high-powered vacuum cleaner (but avoid emptying the vacuum cleaner bag near anyone who suffers from eczema or asthma).
- Ventilate the room regularly and keep the bedrooms cool at night.
- Damp-dust regularly by wiping any surfaces which might collect dust with a damp cloth (for example, windowsills and skirting boards) – this avoids spreading the mites and their faeces into the air.
- Remove feather pillow and quilts and replace them with synthetic ones.
- Consider purchasing anti-dust-mite mattress and pillow covers (available at most department stores). When you are sleeping you are in close contact with house dust mites in your bedding for long periods of time. Covers that totally encase the mat-

tress are the most effective. The covers form a barrier between you and your bedding, and can be used under normal cotton sheets, pillow cases and quilt covers.

- Change the bedding at least weekly if you can to remove any dead skin scales. Wash the bedding at 60°C or above to kill the mites and remove their droppings.
- If bunk beds are used, a child with eczema/asthma should avoid sleeping on the bottom bunk, where exposure to house dust mites will be greater.
- All children have a favourite toy or comforter, which they can take to bed and love. If a child has eczema, it is important that these toys are washed frequently whenever possible. If you are unable to wash the toys, put them inside a plastic bag and put them in the freezer overnight. The cold temperature will kill the house dust mites. Try to keep the number of toys in the room to a minimum.
- Use blinds or curtains that can be washed regularly.
- Vinyl flooring, plain floorboards or cork tiles are easier to clean and can be wiped with a damp cloth. Most houses have carpets in the bedrooms; if it is not practical to remove these then try to vacuum daily if possible and keep your child out of the room when cleaning if he or she suffers from eczema or asthma.

Q. We will be decorating my son's bedroom soon. How can I change things to help his eczema?

If you have the opportunity to change your son's room this is an ideal time to think about taking measures that may reduce the numbers of house dust mites and provide an environment which he will find more comfortable. The key is to minimize the amount of soft furnishing, soft toys and carpets in the room. These provide an ideal environment for the house dust mite. These measures can all help:

- make sure the room is well ventilated
- remove soft furnishings and carpets
- reduce the number of soft toys in the room
- fit blinds at the windows or curtains that can be washed regularly
- use bedding that can be washed at high temperatures

- fit anti-house-dust-mite covers on the bed
- ideally have a heating system which can be regulated
- consider having a fan during the summer (take care with very young children).

Q. I am expecting a new baby. If I reduce the levels of house dust mite in my home will this reduce the chance of my baby developing atopic eczema?

A number of research studies have looked at the question of whether avoidance of house dust mites during pregnancy and early childhood may reduce the number of children who go on to develop atopic eczema. Unfortunately, the results from these different trials have again been conflicting, with no clear benefit being yet proven. Until more research becomes available it is sensible to follow any avoidance measures above that you find practical as part of your lifestyle. Avoidance of house dust mites is most likely to be beneficial if there is a family history of atopic diseases such as eczema, asthma or hayfever. If you are redecorating a nursery this is the ideal time to provide the best environment for your baby – consider laminate flooring and blinds rather than carpets and curtains.

Water quality

The role of water quality in the development of atopic eczema has been recently investigated in a Nottingham-based study. This study showed that atopic eczema was around 50 per cent more common in primary-school children living in areas with hard water when compared with children in areas with soft water. So water quality does seem to play a contributing role. This may be related to the fact that hard water contains substances such as calcium and magnesium which could potentially irritate the skin and lower the threshold for developing eczema, or worsen established eczema. Furthermore, people in areas with hard water often need to use more soaps and cleansing products to produce a good lather when washing, so it may simply be the increased soap use that causes the higher rates of eczema in these areas. Further research studies are currently under way to investigate the link with water quality in more detail. The role of hard and soft water in other types of eczema such as discoid eczema and asteatotic eczema is unknown although it could possibly play a part for the above reasons.

Q. I have atopic eczema. Should I buy a water softener?

As yet there is not enough evidence to recommend that eczema sufferers rush out and buy a water softener – they are expensive and might not help your skin. It is hoped that further studies will clarify their usefulness. Remember that although water may play a role, many other factors are involved in atopic eczema development. Simply getting a water softener is very unlikely to cure your eczema, although in some cases it may help. If you do decide to purchase one make sure you get a reputable water-softener supplier and good plumber. Water softeners are attached to the mains water supply and are usually small enough to fit under the sink.

Q We live in an area with hard water and my child suffers from atopic eczema. How often should he have a bath or shower?

Irrespective of whether you have hard or soft water, there are no firm rules regarding how often to bathe your child. Each child is an individual and it will depend very much on how bad his or her eczema is and what fits in with the family routine. The general advice would generally be no more than once a day, as the skin can become overdry if washing is done to excess. It is important that washing and cleansing are part of the eczema routine. In addition to reducing the chances of infection, washing and bathing remove previous treatments and clean off any loose skin scales so that further treatments can sink into the skin effectively. Generally, bathing is preferable because it allows full immersion of the skin in the water; however, some children find baths too irritating and like to shower. Bath time should be an enjoyable experience. If your child gets upset, complains of stinging and finds the whole experience too traumatic there is no reason why you can't leave it for a few days until he is able to tolerate bathing more easily.

Soaps and cleansing agents

Over the last twenty to thirty years there has been a significant increase in the use of soaps, bubble baths and shower gels in many developed countries. These cleansing agents often contain surfactants and solvents which remove grease and oils – as well as dirt and sweat – from the skin. By reducing the skin's natural greases they encourage water loss from the skin. This can lead to skin dryness and irritation with repeated use. People without eczema will simply produce more natural grease after using these cleansing products and won't run into problems unless they use them too often. However, in people who are prone to developing eczema (for example, those with a family history of atopy and genes that increase their risk), regular use of these cleansing products is often enough to trigger the development of eczema. Elderly patients whose skin has become naturally drier with age also have a lower threshold for developing eczema (for example, asteatotic eczema – see Chapter 1) because of regular use of soaps and bubble baths. By damaging the barrier function of the skin, all of these cleansing products can make it easier for other potentially harmful substances such as house dust mites to get into the skin and exacerbate the eczema.

Q. Can I use soaps, bubble baths and shower gels at all if I have eczema?

It is best to try to avoid conventional soaps and bath/shower gels if you have eczema. People with eczema are much more susceptible to the drying effects of soap, and their skin will feel tight after washing, and become more red and itchy. Bubble baths and shower gels can have a similar drying effect and often contain fragrances (perfumes) and other additives which can irritate the skin. Try to get into the habit of using an emollient as a soap substitute instead (see Chapter 5) for washing, bathing and showering whenever possible. Occasionally people with eczema find that they can use a non-perfumed neutral pH soap providing it doesn't make their eczema flare up.

Q. Can I use baby wipes?

As with other cleansing agents it is not advisable to use baby wipes for children with eczema or for those at high risk of developing eczema. Their skin is far more susceptible to irritation from the surfactants, alcohol and other chemicals in the baby wipes, so cotton wool and water with an emollient soap substitute is generally more suitable.

Q. Can shampoos cause eczema? My daughter has atopic eczema and is always scratching her head but I don't know which shampoo is safe.

The scalp is often affected in people with atopic eczema and it is very unlikely that shampoos are causing the condition. However, they can sometimes make eczema worse in the same way that other harsh cleansing products can exacerbate eczema on the rest of the body. Very occasionally you can develop a contact allergic eczema to chemicals in the shampoo although this is rare and normally produces lots of redness and itching around the hairline skin of the forehead and neck. There are many shampoos available for people with eczema but often a gentle baby shampoo is all that is needed – the key is to keep things simple. Ordinary shampoos can sometimes irritate the scalp so try to stick to non-fragranced products. A number of tar-based shampoos are available for scaly scalps – these can sometimes help but children often complain of the smell. If your daughter has active eczema on her scalp with itchy red scaly skin as opposed to just mild dryness then your doctor can prescribe a steroid scalp preparation such as a gel or mousse (see Chapter 6). It is also important to check that there is no other cause for the itching, such as head lice or scalp ringworm as these are common among school-age children. Get your doctor or nurse to check if you are in any doubt.

Q. Could shampoo be causing my seborrhoeic eczema?

There is no proof that shampoos cause seborrhoeic eczema, which is thought to be related to the growth of a common yeast called *malassezia furfur* on the skin. This yeast lives on many people's skin without causing any problems, but people with seborrhoeic eczema seem to react to the yeast and develop eczema. Anti-yeast shampoos are a very useful treatment in this condition (see Chapter 6). In young children with seborrhoeic eczema gentle baby shampoos and scalp emollients are often sufficient, but make sure that you rinse any shampoo off their scalp completely after washing as any left-over residue may cause irritation and increased scaling.

Q. My elderly father has developed troublesome dry skin over his legs and body. Could this be related to the way he washes?

Yes. It sounds like he has developed asteatotic eczema. This is a common type of eczema that may be caused by overuse of soaps and cleansing products in elderly patients. Many elderly people find it hard to get into the bath or shower and wash using a basin instead. Unfortunately, if the soap is not rinsed off completely, which can be difficult with strip-washing, the soap residue can encourage eczema development. Varicose veins and leg swelling can also contribute to eczema on the legs (see gravitational eczema, Chapter 1).

Household cleaning agents

Hygiene levels in modern homes have improved greatly over recent decades, partly as a result of a large increase in the use of household chemicals such as detergents, solvents, polishes and room fragrances. Although these chemicals are very unlikely to be the sole cause of eczema they may contribute to disease development by causing skin irritation and damage to the skin's barrier function. This in turn may allow other contributing factors to affect the skin more easily. More research is needed to fully assess the role of these products, but in the meantime try to keep their use to a minimum.

Q. My child has atopic eczema. I am worried about using bathroom cleaners in case he reacts to them. Do you have any practical advice to give me for cleaning the bath and house generally?

The bath and shower can be cleaned well with hot soapy water. Providing they are rinsed off and dried properly this shouldn't cause your child any problems. Remember that many eczema creams and bath additives are very greasy and can build up in the bath or shower along with old skin debris unless you clean regularly. This could increase the risk of skin infection and, if very greasy products are used, potentially block drains. Elsewhere in the house try to damp-dust regularly, and rinse surfaces carefully after using any harsh cleaning agents. Avoid polishes, room fragrances and air fresheners, and whenever possible make sure your child is playing in a different room when you are cleaning.

Q. I have been working as a domestic cleaner for 18 months and have developed dreadful eczema on my hands. Is this likely to be have been caused by the cleaning products?

Yes. Cleaning products can strip your hands of moisture and cause an irritant contact dermatitis (see Chapter 1), which is the likely cause of your problem. Even having your hands in and out of water regularly can cause this type of eczema. Cleaning products and rubber gloves can also cause a contact allergy although this is less common. See your doctor to arrange patch-testing (see Chapter 11) if necessary.

Q. I have recently had a baby and I have started getting itchy spots and scaling on my hands. How can I look after my hands with all the extra housework I am doing?

New mothers often find that all the extra washing and cleaning they find themselves doing is enough to trigger eczema. Try these simple tips first.

- Protect your hands from direct contact with soaps and detergents by wearing waterproof, cotton-lined gloves.
- When washing your hands, use lukewarm water and a soap substitute (emollient). All soaps are irritating. No soap is 'gentle to your skin' despite what it might claim.
- Rings often worsen dermatitis by trapping irritating materials beneath them. Remove your rings when doing housework and before washing your hands.
- Protect your hands with an emollient even when your eczema has healed. It can take a long time for your skin to recover completely, and unless you're careful the problem will recur.

If the problem persists see your GP to discuss further treatments or investigations such as patch-testing.

Washing powders

One of the first things people tend to blame when they develop eczema is their washing powder. Comments include 'But I haven't changed my washing powder so why have I developed eczema?', or 'I've tried changing to a non-biological powder and my eczema still hasn't got better'. In actual fact there is very little medical evidence that washing powders, whether biological or non-biological, play a major role in eczema. Washing powders contain a number of substances that could potentially irritate the skin such as surfactants, weak bleaching agents and enzymes (biological powders), but in practice these rarely cause problems provided the clothes are rinsed properly. Rinsing is very important, particularly if you are hand-washing because detergent residue can easily get left on clothes and trigger or worsen your eczema.

Q. Can you recommend any specific washing powder?

No, because what suits one person often doesn't suit another. There is no good evidence to suggest that any one form of detergent – powder, tablet or liquid – is better than another, and a recent small study found no difference in eczema severity between patients using biological and non-biological products. Try to find a product that suits the whole family. Many people with eczema prefer one of the wide range of washing powders now marketed for people with sensitive skin, but many others get on better with standard brands. Use the right amount of product as recommended in the instructions, and remember that you will need to use less in areas with soft water. Generally, biological products are more effective at removing greasy emollients, so if you are using lots of greasy preparations they may actually be more suitable, providing they don't irritate your skin.

Q. Do I need a special washing machine?

No, but it is very important to have an efficient rinse and spin cycle on your washing machine, which will ensure no detergent residue is left in the washing. You may need to do an extra rinse cycle to make sure that no traces of detergent are left on the clothes. Avoid overloading the machine as this will stop the clothes getting rinsed properly. In households with one or more family members suffering from eczema the increased amount of laundry can take a toll on your washing machine. Some people have found that having an extended service warranty, although an added expense initially, does help long term with replacement parts. In particular, greasy emollients can build up and damage the rubber seal. Try running an empty wash on a hot cycle (90°C) once a month using a biological powder – this will help break down the grease and reduce the chance of your seal breaking. If you usually avoid biological powders run another empty wash without powder afterwards to clear the machine.

Q. Can fabric conditioners cause eczema?
As with washing powders, it is unlikely that fabric conditioners (fabric softeners) are a major cause of eczema but they may trigger or worsen the condition in some people. They contain surfactants, fragrances, preservatives and colours, all of which may irritate the skin. Some people can tolerate the newer fabric softeners designed for sensitive skins (often labelled as hypoallergenic) but it is advisable to avoid them completely if you suffer from eczema or have a child at high risk of developing the condition.

Clothing

Some types of clothing can make eczema worse, but generally clothing is not thought to be a major cause in the development of eczema. The roughness of clothing textiles is probably more significant than the type of textile fibre (synthetic or natural), as studies have found that polyester and cotton of similar textile fineness seemed to be equally well tolerated by people with eczema.

Q. Should I stick to cotton clothing if I have eczema?
Cotton clothing is one of the best textiles for eczema sufferers, as wool and synthetic materials often irritate the skin and increase the urge to scratch. Many people can comfortably tolerate cotton/polyester mixed textiles. Again, individuals differ, and you will soon find what suits you best. Many companies provide cotton clothing specifically marketed for people with eczema but do shop around; many of the large superstores/supermarkets also have a wide choice of products. Avoid rough inside seams or labels that may rub on the skin, and ensure that the garments can be washed at 60°C.

Pets

Animals with furry coats shed their hair and skin around the house. Particles in the hair and skin (or in the animal's saliva) can irritate the skin or cause an allergic reaction. Many people with atopic eczema have raised IgE antibody levels to common pets such as cats and dogs, indicating sensitization or allergy to these animals. The fur and saliva of pets can trigger or worsen both eczema and asthma in these individuals (and sometimes also in people without raised IgE levels). Pets also increase the number of skin scales in the house, which in turn can lead to a rise in the levels of house dust mite and further exacerbate your eczema. As with house dust mites, it is not always easy to predict who is most at risk from pets using allergy tests (see Chapter 11). This means that the decision to keep a family pet or not can be extremely difficult, especially as they can be an important source of comfort and friendship.

Q. We have had a dog for over eight years. My daughter has now developed atopic eczema. Should we get rid of our pet?

This is a difficult decision. If your child's eczema clearly gets worse after close contact with the dog or if she develops any other symptoms such as hives (urticaria) or wheezing after being in the room with the animal then it is wise to consider giving your pet to another home. Remember, however, that following removal of animals from the home it may take many months for the remnants of fur and saliva to decrease because of widespread distribution in carpets and soft furnishings. This means that your child's symptoms may not improve immediately. If you are unsure whether the dog is making her symptoms worse then discuss allergy testing with your doctor (see Chapter 11). A negative allergy test makes it unlikely that the dog is playing a major role but does not completely exclude allergy. Furthermore, even if your child is not truly allergic to your dog, having an animal around may indirectly make her eczema worse by increasing the level of house dust mites in your home. If you decide to keep the pet then make sure you vacuum regularly, keep the dog out of the bedrooms and put a washable sheet on any furniture that your dog sits on.

It is generally advisable not to get a pet if there is a strong family history of atopy, although research on the exact role of pets in causing eczema is still very limited and further studies are currently in progress. Not getting a pet in the first place is a lot easier than facing the hard decision of whether to get rid of your pet later on. The timing of exposure to pets may be very significant. Some studies suggest that exposure to pets in early life is most likely to trigger allergy, so it's probably wise not to get a pet until your children are older if eczema, asthma or hayfever run in the family.

Q. When my daughter goes to her friend's house she always comes back very itchy. They have a cat and a dog. Should I stop her from going?

It sounds likely that your daughter is allergic to the pets, but you don't want to stop her seeing her friends. Taking some simple precautions may help to prevent her skin from flaring up.

- Suggest she avoids direct animal contact or otherwise wears cotton gloves when handling/stroking the pets.
- Apply an emollient before she visits her friend's house. Wash the emollient off when she gets home, then reapply another layer of emollient to keep her skin moist and cool.
- Ask your doctor about antihistamine tablets if she is getting hives on her skin, itchy eyes or a runny nose during visits to her friend's house (see Chapter 11).

Temperature

Over the last fifty years the number of houses with central heating, double-glazing and cavity-wall insulation has increased dramatically, resulting in a significant rise in the average indoor temperature and in humidity and dampness. Over this time the number of people suffering with atopic eczema has also risen substantially. In atopic eczema temperature and humidity changes may partly contribute to the condition by encouraging high levels of house dust mite in the home. However, extremes of temperature can also directly worsen atopic eczema. Temperature and humidity may also be important in many other types of eczema such as asteatotic eczema, pompholyx eczema, discoid eczema and contact eczema.

Q. My child gets very hot in bed and this seems to make his eczema worse. How can I keep him cool?

At bedtime children often find they get very hot and start to scratch. Keeping the room at a comfortable temperature level is very important – if the heating is on keep it low, open a window and don't have the bed near direct heat. In bed your child may find wearing two layers of thin clothing better than wearing one thick layer. He will then be able to add or remove these layers in order to regulate his own comfort levels. Some children also get on better with several layers of bedding such as cotton sheets and blankets rather than a duvet. If your child prefers a duvet try using two lighter duvets rather than a winter-thickness duvet – again, this will allow him to kick one off if he is too hot. Many parents apply emollients too thickly at bedtime, hoping it will last longer. Unfortunately this can sometimes have an adverse effect and make the child too hot, so try using a thinner layer if over-heating is a problem.

Q. Do changes in temperature make eczema worse? If so, what can I do to help my child?

Yes, changes in temperature do make eczema worse. Again, each person is different, but the skin of children with eczema is particularly susceptible to extremes of temperature. In the summer they often find that if they become hot and sweaty their skin gets worse. In the winter months, the combination of cold, frosty and windy weather outside and central heating indoors can have a drying and irritating effect on the skin. In the summer months the use of a lighter emollient (moisturizer) may help, because many of the heavier greasier emollients can add to the overheating. During the colder months a heavier emollient can help to protect the skin when exposed to the harsh weather.

Q. I get attacks of blistering eczema on my hands which is always worse in the summer, especially when I've spent lots of time outdoors. Is this related to the heat?

It sounds like you are getting pompholyx eczema. This type of eczema can be triggered by heat and sweating, although a primary cause is often never found. Occasionally, contact allergies to plants can cause hand blistering in the summer months. Discuss the problem with your GP, who can arrange patch-testing (see Chapter 11) if a contact allergy is suspected.

Pollution

Higher levels of atopic eczema have been shown in people living close (under 50 metres) to busy roads, although the importance of outdoor pollution has not been confirmed in all studies. High levels of sulphur dioxide, nitrous oxides and diesel particles from car emissions can potentially irritate the skin and may lower the threshold for developing eczema or worsen established eczema. Pollution can also play a role in asthma. However, the exact role of outdoor pollution in causing atopic eczema, as well as its role in other types of eczema, remains to be confirmed in further studies. Tobacco smoke and gas fumes from cooking have been implicated in contributing to atopic eczema development in some studies, but again the role of indoor pollution remains to be confirmed by further research.

Pollen and moulds

Raised IgE levels to grass or tree pollen are very common in people with atopic eczema. However, pollen does not make most people's atopic eczema worse. It appears to be much more important in triggering asthma and hayfever (which many eczema patients also suffer from) as it is airborne and enters the nose and lungs easily. Most people with atopic eczema find their skin is not really affected by the pollen season, and actually usually improves in the spring and summer months when pollen levels are at their highest. This improvement is often caused by the effects of natural sunlight. If your eczema does get worse in the pollen season then keep the windows shut in the early morning and evening when pollen levels are at their highest, and apply liberal amounts of emollient before going outside. When you get back indoors wash the emollient off and reapply it to get rid of any pollen particles that may have stuck on to your skin. Certain moulds can also be found in the air, especially during the summer months, but their role in causing eczema has not been well proven.

Dietary factors

People frequently wonder whether something in their diet is causing their eczema. It is tempting to want to blame something you are eating, especially if you think you may be able to clear your skin up by simple changes to your diet. Unfortunately, it is rarely that simple.

The role of diet has been most extensively studied in patients with atopic eczema, and dietary factors are not thought to play a significant role in other types of eczema. The rise in atopic eczema over the last fifty years has been associated with significant changes in people's diets, especially in Westernized countries. People now consume a much wider variety of foods which could potentially cause allergies. More varied diets are also often introduced at a much younger age than previously. This has stimulated lots of research to see if foods really are a common cause of eczema. To summarize the results of these studies:

- if you become allergic or intolerant to certain foods they can cause or worsen your atopic eczema although this appears to be uncommon in the majority of people
- food is most likely to be an important factor in causing eczema in a small subset of children less than three years of age
- the most common foods to cause allergy are cow's milk, egg, nuts (peanuts and treenuts), fish, soya and wheat
- food allergies are usually immediate-type allergies (see Chapter 11) which produce hives (urticaria) in the skin, although subsequent development or worsening of eczema (delayed type allergy) can also occur
- allergy tests are not always good at predicting whether your diet is causing or exacerbating your eczema. The best way of proving whether diet is important to you as an individual is to eliminate the food for six to eight weeks although this will usually require the supervision of a dietician (essential in young children).

For more information on food allergies in people with established eczema see Chapter 11.

Q. My first child has atopic eczema. Should I avoid any foods when I am pregnant or breastfeeding to reduce the chance of my next baby developing eczema?
It is now thought that babies can be exposed to substances that can trigger allergy (allergens) before they are born, and that these

allergens *may* affect their chances of developing eczema or allergies in childhood. These allergens get into the mother's bloodstream from things she has eaten or inhaled, and are passed to the baby through the placenta. Researchers are currently looking at whether changes in the mother's diet and lifestyle during pregnancy or breastfeeding can reduce the development of allergies in their children. Doctors and healthcare professionals currently recommend that mothers exclusively breastfeed their babies for six months if possible, as formula feeds contain cow's milk. Many studies have suggested that exclusive breastfeeding in this way may reduce your baby's chances of developing atopy or food allergies. Remember that breast milk provides all your baby's nutritional needs for the first six months of life, and also has other protective properties which can reduce your baby's chances of developing infections.

It is currently advised that peanuts are avoided by pregnant or breastfeeding women if they, their partner or any of their children suffer from diagnosed allergy or atopy. If you have a strong family history of allergies or atopic diseases (such as atopic eczema, asthma or hayfever) there is also some evidence that avoiding foods such as milk and eggs while pregnant or breastfeeding may reduce the risk of your baby developing atopic eczema. However, this evidence is limited and such diets are not routinely recommended. If you wish to consider pursuing this further, see your doctor, who can arrange for you to see a dietician. It is very important that breastfeeding mothers eat enough protein, calcium and vitamins, and it is very easy to become deficient in these nutrients if a dietician is not involved.

Q. What if I can't breastfeed my baby?

If there is a strong history of allergy in the family and it is not possible for you to breastfeed you should discuss with your doctor or health visitor whether a hydrolysed formula (milk hydrolysate) may be suitable. Hydrolysed formulas contain cow's milk but the milk proteins are broken down into a more simplified form that is less likely to cause allergy. They are generally used for babies at very high risk of developing atopy (both parents and/or a brother or sister who are atopic). Hydrolysed formulas can also be tried if your baby's eczema develops or worsens after introducing standard formula bottle feeds. Soya milk is another alternative to cow's milk formula but can cause allergies so it is not recommended for the prevention of eczema.

Q. I will be weaning my baby soon. What should I think about when planning her meals to reduce her chance of developing atopic eczema?

Current guidance in the UK for mothers is that they should delay introducing solid foods until the baby is six months old. If there is a history of eczema or allergy in the family it is sensible to start with foods that are least likely to cause allergy, such as baby rice, pure fruits and vegetables. Introduce one food at a time, giving it daily for one week before you decide whether it has an adverse effect (skin rash or loose watery stools). If you observe an immediate reaction such as swelling and redness of the lips and face, seek medical advice before trying it again. It is best to avoid peanuts for at least three years if there is a family history of allergy. Both you and your baby should have a good, well-balanced diet, and if restricted diets are used you should always ask to be referred to a dietician for further advice.

Reduced exposure to infection

In contrast to many diseases, exposure to certain types of infection is actually thought to have a beneficial role in preventing atopic eczema development. Although all the causes of atopic eczema are not fully understood, one of the most common hypotheses is that reduced exposure to infection in early life increases the risk of developing the condition. This theory is known as the 'hygiene hypothesis' and has arisen from the observation that the rise in atopic eczema over recent years has paralleled a dramatic reduction in infectious diseases.

Q. How could improved hygiene possibly cause atopic eczema?

Your immune system contains white blood cells called T-helper lymphocytes (or T-cells). These can be divided into two types – type 1 (Th1) and type 2 (Th2). The blood of people with atopic eczema contains higher levels of Th2 lymphocytes than normal and these cells are thought to contribute to atopic eczema development. People without atopic eczema have higher levels of Th1 cells.

In the womb and for a short period after birth healthy people produce high levels of Th2 cells. As your immune system matures with age the level of Th2 cells should go down and the levels of Th1 cells should go up – this is part of normal development. In order for this normal maturation to take place your body needs to be exposed to common infections in the environment early on in your life. These infections stimulate a rise in Th1 cells. If you don't get exposed to common childhood infections this seems to stop your immune system from developing properly and you keep high levels of Th2 cells. This Th1/Th2 imbalance is then thought to cause atopic eczema.

Q. What evidence is there to support this theory?

Studies on blood samples have demonstrated that these changes in T-lymphocytes do appear to be important. There is also good evidence from epidemiological studies that atopic eczema is more common in smaller families, in children without brothers and sisters, and in children who don't attend nurseries. All of these children will have had less exposure to cross infection from other children. One recent study showed that the risk of developing atopic eczema was nearly 50 per cent lower in children who had their first chest infection before the age of six months. Some studies have also shown that children brought up on farms have a reduced risk of developing atopic diseases, which may be related to increased exposure to infection early on in life.

Q. Why are babies born with high Th2 levels?

Th2 cells don't just cause atopic eczema – they actually play an important role in fighting parasite infections such as intestinal worms. Parasite infections are now extremely uncommon in Westernized countries but the raised Th2 cells at birth seem to have been retained through evolution.

Q. So what does the hygiene hypothesis mean for people with atopic eczema?

So far the hygiene hypothesis remains a theory although there is strong evidence to support it as a cause of eczema. The hygiene hypothesis applies to developmental changes very early on in life and so if you already have atopic eczema it probably won't alter the management of your disease at all. However, for babies at high risk of developing atopic eczema it would seem sensible to encourage mixing with other children as much as possible, particularly in the first few months of life. Research being done currently is looking at ways of exposing high-risk infants to controlled doses of infection either in the womb or early on in life. Such approaches include giving safe bacteria by mouth (probiotics – see Chapter 10) or by injection (*mycobacterial vaccae* injections), although at present these interventions are still experimental.

Q. If normal childhood infections are thought to be beneficial then is it still OK for my child to have his routine immunizations?

Yes, it is very important that you give your child all the recommended immunizations (vaccines) as normal. The only reason to delay your child's immunizations is if he is being treated with certain ointments (see Chapter 7) or tablet treatment to suppress his immune system (see Chapter 9), or if he is having a bad flare-up of his eczema. If your child has severe egg allergy, you need to discuss immunization with your GP (see Chapter 11).

There is currently no evidence that any of the immunizations recommended by the Department of Health will increase your child's risk of developing eczema, or worsen established eczema. Furthermore, children who are not vaccinated run the risk of severe or long-term health damage if they do catch the diseases that they have not been protected against. Routine immunizations are designed to protect your child (and others who may come into contact with them) from potentially dangerous infections, and not from the more common childhood viral and bacterial infections such as coughs, colds and impetigo. Vaccinated children will still get plenty of exposure to less harmful and potentially beneficial infections throughout their childhood.

Gravity

Gravity is an important cause of gravitational eczema, but it doesn't play a significant role in causing other types of eczema.

Gravity increases the pressure in your leg veins. If the pressure in the leg veins becomes too great the sluggish flow of blood causes fluid to collect up under the skin and trigger eczema. When you are young your leg veins are very efficient at counteracting the effects of gravity, but over time the veins can become weaker. Varicose veins and previous deep vein thromboses (blood clots) increase your risk of developing gravitational eczema.

Q. I have varicose veins and if I have been on my legs for a long time my ankles swell and I get an itchy rash. How can I stop the swelling from happening?

You can help to reduce the swelling in your legs by not standing still for long periods. Regular exercise will definitely help. This is because when you exercise your leg, muscles help to squeeze blood up your veins. Exercise can also help you shed a few pounds if you are overweight, and this will reduce the pressure in your legs even more. Try to walk to work or up the stairs rather than sitting on a bus or standing in lifts. When you are sitting down try to get your feet elevated whenever you can, ideally above your hips or higher. Wearing compression stockings in the day will also help the swelling in your legs, and reduce the chance of you getting gravitational eczema. Lightweight support stockings can be bought from some pharmacies and department stores. Some people will benefit from tighter compression stockings, which your GP can prescribe if appropriate – discuss this with your GP if the problem persists. Occasionally varicose vein surgery can help but not always. Your GP may refer you to your local vascular surgeon to discuss whether surgery is an option for you. The surgeon may organize a special ultrasound picture (called a duplex scan) of your leg veins to show the blood flow in more detail – this can give useful information about whether surgery is likely to help or not.

Stress

It is well recognized that emotional stress can contribute to the development of eczema, although stress is a difficult topic to study accurately as it is very subjective. All the types of eczema discussed in Chapter 1 can potentially be made worse by severe emotional stresses such as chronic depression, bereavement, job changes, moving house or getting married. It is not uncommon for adult patients to present with eczema for the first time after a period of stress. Although stress is rarely the primary cause of eczema, it certainly seems to lower the threshold for developing the condition, and often makes established eczema flare up temporarily. Emotional stresses are discussed in more detail in Chapter 14.

Chapter 3
Eczema and infections

Infections can be caused by bacteria, viruses and fungi, all of which are common in the environment and are easily spread between individuals. They can affect your eczema in many different ways, and it is important to recognize them because they can often make your eczema worse. Although many of the infections discussed below are more common in children, they can affect people of all ages and all different types of eczema. Infections can involve the whole of your body (general infections), or may just affect the skin as a consequence of your underlying eczema (secondary infections).

General infections

Common viral infections such as chickenpox, measles, flu and the common cold are probably no more prevalent in people with eczema than in people without it. These infections may make your eczema flare up although many people actually find their eczema improves temporarily. At the moment there is no good evidence to suggest that any particular infection will make eczema worse or better, and the flare-ups and clear periods after infections may simply be because of the variable nature of your underlying eczema. Similarly, there is no evidence that any of the common childhood vaccinations will make eczema worse and these should not be withheld from your child (see page 42).

Secondary infections

Secondary infections refer to skin infections that develop on top of your underlying eczema. A normal healthy skin is important to defend our bodies from bacteria and viruses in the environment. In eczema the skin is damaged and cracked, and doesn't act as a good barrier. Bacteria and viruses can get into your skin much more easily if you suffer from eczema, and can also spread more quickly. Secondary infection is always important to exclude whenever your eczema flares badly for no obvious reason.

Bacterial infections

Bacteria are microscopic organisms that are invisible to the naked eye. The most important type of bacteria in people with eczema is *Staphylococcus aureus*. Known as *Staph. aureus*, it can be found on the skin of 5 to 20 per cent of people without eczema, but usually in low amounts. In contrast, it can be found in over 90 per cent of people with inflamed eczema, and is one of the most common causes of secondary skin infection. Another type of bacteria, called *Streptococcus*, can also cause secondary skin infections in people with eczema, but it is less common.

Q. So when do bacteria actually cause problems?

The amount of *Staph. aureus* on your skin is roughly proportional to the severity of your eczema. In mild eczema only very low levels of bacteria are found. At these low levels the bacteria are probably simply colonizing the skin – this means that they are living on the skin without causing much of a problem. However, when the levels of bacteria increase they will start to make your eczema worse, and this is called bacterial infection. Eczema that has become infected with bacteria is sometimes called impetiginized eczema – this is because the same bacteria cause a common childhood skin infection called impetigo (see below).

Q. How do I know when my skin is infected?

Infected eczema is usually wet and weepy, with yellow crusty patches or open oozing areas of skin. Small blisters filled with yellowish-white pus may develop on the eczema. Your skin will feel more red and sore than usual and you may also feel generally unwell or even have a temperature, although this is not always the case.

Q. How do the bacteria make my eczema worse?

Bacterial infection causes direct inflammation of the skin which produces redness and swelling. Bacteria are also thought to aggravate eczema indirectly by producing toxins called exotoxins. These toxins can activate the cells in your immune system (T-cells) that play a key role in eczema development. The toxins act as superantigens, which are substances that can activate many

T-cells in your immune system at the same time to cause a whole cascade of immune reactions that produce even more skin inflammation. Bacteria may also cause skin irritation from proteins in their cell wall or enzymes that they produce. All these factors will make your eczema worse.

Q. How is bacterial infection treated?

If you suspect infection you should go to your doctor as early as possible. If your eczema is weepy and crusty your doctor will usually prescribe a course of oral antibiotics (syrup or tablets) for one to two weeks. Your doctor or nurse may take a skin swab (using a special cotton bud) to make a culture of the bacteria, although in most cases *Staph. aureus* will be the bacteria responsible. Flucloxacillin is one of the most common antibiotics used to treat *Staph. aureus* infection. If swabs show *Streptococcal* infection, penicillin is usually prescribed. Erythromycin is useful in people who are allergic to penicillin. If the infection doesn't respond to antibiotic treatment a skin swab should always be taken. This will tell your doctor which bacteria are causing the infection and the best antibiotic medicine to use.

Q. Will antibiotics help my eczema even when it isn't weepy or crusty?

Research studies have looked at whether oral antibiotics are of any benefit in eczema that isn't obviously infected, and have found no evidence that they help significantly. If your eczema is dry and scaly with very little redness or swelling in the skin, the low levels of bacteria present will usually clear with the standard creams and ointments prescribed for your eczema. As the treatments restore your skin barrier to normal, the colonizing bacteria also decrease.

Q. Should I continue with my steroid ointment if I have infected eczema?

Yes, it is important to treat the underlying eczema as well as the infection. Although steroids by themselves can encourage the spread of infections, providing you are also being treated with antibiotics this will cover the infection effectively.

Q. My GP has given me a steroid cream which contains an antibiotic. Should I use this long term to keep the bacteria levels on my skin down?

Steroid/antibiotic combination creams or ointments (see Chapter 6) are often prescribed for localized or mildly infected eczema. Although not much research evidence exists to show that these combined preparations are better than plain topical steroids for infected or non-infected eczema, many patients do find them useful for a short course of one to two weeks when their eczema flares up. There is some evidence that a two-week course of an antibiotic ointment called mupirocin (Bactroban®) can help eczema when used along with a steroid ointment. However, there are serious concerns that widespread use topical antibiotic creams and ointments (especially mupirocin) may encourage bacteria to become resistant to these antibiotics over time (see below). Very occasionally antibiotic creams can also cause skin irritation or allergy and actually make your eczema worse, although this is rare.

If your GP does recommend a topical steroid/antibiotic combination it should usually be used for a maximum of two weeks to clear the infection, and not for maintenance treatment. In widespread secondarily infected eczema, oral antibiotics and topical steroids are the treatment of choice.

Q. What is antibiotic resistance?

Antibiotic resistance occurs when bacteria develop mechanisms to avoid being killed by antibiotics. Resistance is an increasing problem worldwide and usually develops when antibiotics have been used for prolonged periods. When bacteria develop antibiotic resistance they no longer respond to standard courses of antibiotics and can become very difficult to treat. With increasing numbers of antibiotic-resistant bacteria in the environment this will not only cause problems for people with skin infections (such as infected eczema) but also for people with more serious internal infections. The increasing use of topical steroids that contain the antibiotic fusidic acid (for example, Fucidin H® and Fucibet®) for the maintenance treatment of eczema has been linked to rising levels of fusidic acid resistance in many parts of the UK. One of the reasons that mupirocin is not widely used to treat infected eczema is that it is very useful in the treatment of methicillin-resistant *Staph. aureus* (MRSA) – a strain of *Staph. aureus* that is resistant to many other antibiotics. Widespread use of mupirocin would potentially lead to the development of increased resistance to this antibiotic and limit its usefulness in many other areas of medicine. Short courses of topical antibiotic therapy (for less than two weeks) are much less likely to result in the emergence of resistant bacteria.

Q. There has been an outbreak of impetigo at my daughter's nursery. Could this make her atopic eczema worse?

Yes. Impetigo is an infectious bacterial skin condition which is common in otherwise healthy children and is also usually caused by *Staph. aureus*. Impetigo starts as small, superficial, fragile blisters which burst easily and then start to weep and produce golden yellow crust. It can affect any area of the body but most often involves the face. Impetigo can spread between children very easily, so children are usually kept out of school or nursery until they have been treated with oral antibiotics or antibiotic creams. Children with eczema are particularly prone to catching the infection and developing impetiginized eczema, so you will need to be extra vigilant and report any sign of your daughter's eczema flaring to your doctor.

Q. Can scalded skin syndrome affect people with eczema?

Scalded skin syndrome is a rare condition that is caused by bacterial infection with certain strains of *Staph. aureus*. It tends to occur in young children and can affect those with or without eczema, although people with eczema are at higher risk because of their damaged skin. The strains of *Staph. aureus* responsible for the condition produce a toxin which is released throughout the body. This toxin causes the skin to become red and peel off, so affected children look like they have been scalded. The problem usually starts in moist skin folds such as the nappy area or armpits. Sometimes the 'scalded' skin remains just in the skin creases. At other times it can spread to the whole body. In many cases the affected child may have had a little patch of impetigo or infected eczema beforehand. The skin may be blistered and become very tender and hot. You may also notice that the skin peels and looks dirty at the edges. Peeling is often more notice-able on the palms and soles because the skin is thicker there. The child may be miserable and have a temperature.

It is important to recognize scalded skin syndrome because oral (or sometimes intravenous) antibiotics are needed. Children usually make an excellent recovery despite the alarming appear-ance, and fortunately it is usually a one-off problem.

Q. How can I prevent my child's eczema from becoming infected in the future?

One of the most important things is not to allow your child's skin to dry out. Cracked and broken skin creates an ideal home for *Staph aureus*. Regular use of an emollient may help to dis-courage the infection. If your child has frequent episodes of infected eczema, then try using an emollient with an added anti-septic (see Chapter 5). Some children and adults have a reservoir of bacteria in their noses and this can cause recurrent infections. A skin swab from the nostrils can confirm if this is the case, and an antibiotic ointment can be used to clear the bacteria. Family members may also need to be swabbed. You should discuss this further with your doctor or nurse.

Q. If my eczema becomes infected can I pass the infection on to other people?

If you have infected eczema you should use separate towels and flannels to reduce the risk of the bacteria spreading. It is very important to wash your hands after contact with the infected skin. Children should be kept off school until treatment has been started and the infection is starting to clear.

Viral infections

Viruses are microscopic organisms that can cause a number of common diseases ranging from chickenpox to the common cold. The most important viruses to affect people with eczema are the herpes virus and certain types of wart virus as discussed below. These viral infections are mainly a problem in people with atopic eczema.

Eczema herpeticum

The cold-sore virus (*herpes simplex*) can spread very rapidly in people with atopic eczema and this is called eczema herpeticum. Although eczema herpeticum is rare, it is a very important secondary infection to recognize because it can potentially be serious. Cold sores are very common in otherwise healthy individuals, especially around the mouth. In people without eczema they usually remain localized to a small area of skin and clear up by themselves over a week or two. However, if the surrounding skin is inflamed and damaged from eczema the cold-sore virus can spread over the whole face or even over the rest of the body.

Q. How can I tell if I have eczema herpeticum and what should I do?

Eczema herpeticum will usually be obvious because it makes your eczema very sore and much worse than usual. In the early stages you will see a lot of small blisters filled with clear fluid surrounded by a bright red halo on the surface of the skin. Within one to two days, these blisters break quickly to leave a lot of small round punched-out sores on the skin. The area may become very painful and you may feel generally unwell, especially if the problem spreads. See your doctor immediately if you suspect eczema herpeticum as a five-day course of antiviral tablets (such as aciclovir) is needed. In severe cases hospital admission is required.

Q. Should I continue with my steroid ointment if I have eczema herpeticum?

Although topical steroids can encourage spread of the herpes virus, so can untreated inflamed eczema. If you have active eczema it is usually safe to continue treatment with your topical steroid once antiviral treatment has been started, but you should discuss this with your doctor first. If you are using Protopic® or Elidel® you should stop these treatments and consult your doctor (see Chapter 7).

Q. How can I avoid catching eczema herpeticum?

It is difficult to avoid the cold-sore virus completely because it is very common in otherwise healthy people. If you have eczema you should avoid close contact with people who have active cold sores. Equally, if your child has eczema do not kiss him or her if you have a cold sore, otherwise you may pass on the cold-sore virus. Once you have been exposed to the herpes virus it remains in the nerves that supply your skin and can become reactivated from time to time, especially if you are run down and stressed. If you do suffer from repeated cold sores (they tend to affect the same place each time), it often helps to treat them quickly with aciclovir cream available from your pharmacy. Aciclovir cream is effective only if applied as soon as the cold sore develops and should never be used to treat established eczema herpeticum as cream alone is not strong enough once the virus has spread. If you are getting cold sores very frequently discuss with your doctor whether a course of low-dose antiviral tablets for several months may be beneficial to try to suppress the attacks.

Chickenpox

Chickenpox is a common general infection in children, whether they have eczema or not. Although chickenpox is caused by a type of herpes virus it doesn't often cause eczema herpeticum like the cold-sore virus does. However, chickenpox does cause a nasty widespread skin rash with plenty of itchy red spots that rapidly turn into small blisters. The virus is usually spread by airborne droplets, and children with chickenpox are infectious to others until all the blisters have crusted over and dried up. Children with chickenpox who also have eczema can continue with their emollients and use aqueous calamine to dry up the blisters provided it does not irritate their eczema. If your child is using topical steroids discuss with your doctor whether these need to be stopped, and if the chickenpox does become severe you should see your doctor immediately. It is absolutely essential to seek urgent medical attention if you or your child develops chickenpox during or shortly after taking any form of immunosuppressant tablet for your eczema (or associated asthma) such as oral steroids or ciclosporin (see Chapter 9) as this can cause the chickenpox virus to become very widespread.

Molluscum contagiosum

Molluscum contagiosum are caused by a common type of wart virus that infects the top layers of the skin. Molluscum develop as small skin-coloured or pink shiny bumps on the skin that often form little clusters – if you look very carefully you often see a small depression or dent in the middle of the bump. They can occur anywhere on the body including the face and genital area. They typically affect children between the ages of four and eight years but anyone including adults can get them. Although molluscum are extremely common in all school-age children they are more common in people who suffer from atopic eczema.

Q. How do molluscum differ from the normal warts that people often get on their hands and feet?

Molluscum look different (much rounder and smoother) and do not usually last as long. They are caused by a different type of wart virus (*pox virus*) from common hand warts (*papilloma virus*). Although molluscum contagiosum are more common in people with eczema, there is not a lot of evidence that common hand and foot warts are any more common in eczema patients than in the general population. Both molluscum and common hand and foot warts usually clear up spontaneously with time.

Q. Why are molluscum contagiosum more common in people with eczema?

Molluscum contagiosum are probably more common in people with eczema because the broken and damaged skin that charac-terizes eczema allows the virus to get into the skin and spread more easily. It is also possible that creams and ointments may encourage molluscum to spread, but it is essential that you con-tinue to use your normal eczema treatments, otherwise the skin will become more damaged. Treat the areas affected by mollus-cum last, and wash your hands before applying creams to other parts of your body.

Q. Are molluscum contagious?

Yes, but only in a mild sense. Direct skin-to-skin contact is needed to spread the virus, and typically this occurs only between young children of a susceptible age. Occasionally, adults get molluscum, but most adults will have had the infection in childhood and be immune to the virus. There is no reason to stop your child from attending school or swimming just because he or she has molluscum.

Q. Are molluscum serious?

Absolutely not. They are a harmless, self-limiting infection of the skin and have nothing to do with any serious internal ill-nesses. Molluscum usually don't bother children at all although they may look a little unpleasant. Quite understandably parents worry because they often don't know what they are or if they will go away of their own accord. Occasionally, they may be itchy or they may bleed when the child scratches them. This should not be a cause for alarm and scratching it may in fact help the virus to disappear more quickly from the skin. Sometimes, one or two of the molluscum may become large and red and look as if they are infected. Usually this swelling and redness is a sign that the body's immune system is getting rid of them naturally, although very occasionally molluscum can become infected. If you are worried, see your doctor, who can prescribe a short course of an antibiotic cream (or tablets) if necessary.

Q. Will molluscum go away?

Yes, the majority of molluscum will disappear within 6 to 18 months although some stubborn ones can last for longer. Typically, a child will have a patch of molluscum on one area of the body. Some disappear as some new ones appear, until even-tually the whole infection burns itself out as the child develops his or her own immunity against the molluscum virus. Once you have developed immunity you are very unlikely to get the infec-tion again later on in life. Children tend to get molluscum more than adults because they have not yet developed their own natural immunity to the virus.

Q. Do molluscum need to be treated?

No, not usually, because they go away of their own accord without leaving a scar. Destructive methods such as freezing them with liquid nitrogen or pricking them and squeezing out the contents can be used, but these are often painful for the child and cause unnecessary distress and sometimes scarring. It is inadvisable to treat children for molluscum unless they are unusually large or persistent and your child is asking for treatment.

Fungal and yeast infections

Fungal and yeast infections do not usually cause secondary infection in people with atopic eczema. However, occasionally a yeast called *candida* (thrush) can secondarily infect eczema in warm, moist sites such as under the breasts or around the genital area. Skin infected with *candida* looks red and sore and may be studded with lots of tiny white pus-filled spots. Treatment with an anti-yeast cream from your doctor or pharmacist will usually clear the problem quickly. A skin yeast called *malassezia furfur* is thought to play a role in seborrhoeic eczema, and anti-yeast creams and shampoos can be very helpful in this condition (see Chapter 6). Ringworm fungus can occasionally develop in people with eczema, and usually starts as athlete's foot. It is important to see your doctor if you suspect this problem as he or she can check your toenails to see if they are also infected. Toenails infected with fungus generally need treatment with antifungal tablets (available on prescription) rather than topical treatment to get rid of the problem effectively.

Chapter 4
General advice on treating eczema

There is a wide variety of very effective treatments for eczema. This is good news because it means that most people can control their condition extremely well using simple therapies once the basic principles of treatment have been explained. The development of new and exciting treatments along with better research into eczema therapy means that you can now be more in control of your skin than ever before. A number of different healthcare professionals are at hand to provide you with the information, education and support you need to overcome the condition and get on with your life. This chapter explains who these people are and how to use them most effectively.

It is important to understand that all the eczema treatments that are currently available are very good at controlling eczema but they won't make it go away for ever. In other words, they won't cure your eczema permanently, because as yet there is no cure. This means that you may need to use the treatments on and off for months, or sometimes years, depending on how long your eczema lasts. Some people are surprised when their eczema comes back and think their treatments haven't worked, but this is not the case. The treatments will work while they are being used but you need to be prepared to use them intermittently until you grow out of your eczema naturally. Fortunately, the treatments are so effective that many people don't notice their eczema at all while they are using them, and often the skin will stay clear for quite some time in between treatments, giving you a long break from your symptoms and helping you get on with your life.

Sources of help

You

To have the best chance of overcoming your eczema you need to be actively involved in treatment from the start. This is very important because eczema treatment revolves around controlling *your* symptoms. Your doctor or nurse will be able to help and advise you when you see them, but *you* are the one who will be treating the eczema on a day-to-day basis, possibly for months or even years. Eczema can change from day to day so to be in control of your skin you need to learn how to change your treatments safely and effectively depending on how good or bad your eczema is. This means learning to use short bursts of stronger treatment when the eczema flares, and stepping down to weaker treatments as it settles for maintenance therapy. Eczema treatment is very individual, and treatments that work for one person might not work as well for another. Get involved in treatment decisions by letting your doctor know what treatments you find most effective or unhelpful. Make sure your doctor has a good idea of how your eczema has been between consultations – keep a diary if necessary.

Treatments can be time-consuming and sometimes messy, and it can take time to see a full improvement in your skin. However, once you get into a treatment routine it does become much easier, and you'll be surprised at what a difference it makes to your skin.

Your general practitioner (GP)

Your GP is the first person to see to discuss treatment. He or she is absolutely essential to guide and oversee your treatment and help tailor it to you as an individual. Remember that everyone's eczema is different and your GP will be able to help you decide which treatment is best for you depending on what the skin looks like and how much the eczema is interfering with your life. Your GP will also be able to prescribe your treatments, and will know how and when to refer you for more specialist help if necessary.

Your practice nurse or health visitor

Many GP surgeries have nurses who work in the surgery who are trained to help you look after your skin once your GP has diagnosed which type of eczema you have. Some practice nurses and health visitors run special eczema clinics – ask your GP if there is one in your area.

A GP with a special interest in dermatology (GPwSI)

GPs need to know a lot about everything and don't treat just skin diseases. They are trained to have a broad knowledge about all diseases, so many GPs have only a short training in the management of skin disease. Some GPs do extra training in how to treat skin diseases because they have a special interest in dermatology. These GPs work in the community in a GP surgery but usually help out in the hospital dermatology clinics on a regular basis to keep up their knowledge. If there is a GP with a special interest in dermatology near you your GP may refer you to him or her for further treatment advice rather than sending you straight to a hospital specialist.

Hospital dermatologist (skin specialist)

Most (but not all) hospitals have a dermatologist who specializes in diagnosing and treating skin diseases. Some big hospitals have large dermatology departments with several dermatologists working together. Smaller hospitals may have just one dermatologist. Wherever you live your GP will be able to refer you to a dermatologist, if necessary, for further advice on treatment, although some people may have to travel further than others to get to their nearest hospital. Only a small proportion of people with eczema need to be referred to a dermatologist as most people can learn how to treat their eczema safely and effectively with simple treatments from their GP. For atopic eczema there are published guidelines for your GP that recommend who should be referred on to see a dermatologist (see box on facing page). For other types of eczema your GP should refer you to see a dermatologist if treatment in primary care (your GP's surgery) fails and the eczema continues to trouble you.

Other hospital specialists

In some hospitals paediatricians (children's doctors) care for children with eczema, especially if the child also has asthma. However, most paediatricians will have had less training in skin-disease management than a dermatologist, and if there is any

Atopic eczema referral guidelines

Referral to a dermatologist is advised if you:

- have severe eczema that has not responded to appropriate treatment from your GP
- have infected eczema (weeping, crusting or pus-filled spots in the eczema) and treatment with an antibiotic by mouth and topical steroid has not worked
- have eczema that is causing severe social or psychological problems
- have eczema that is needing excessive amounts of strong steroid creams or ointments
- have eczema that your GP has not managed to control satisfactorily and is still causing troublesome symptoms
- have eczema that may benefit from specialist advice on how to use the treatments (for example, bandaging techniques)
- have eczema that your GP suspects is caused by a contact allergy and you may need patch-testing (see Chapter 11)
- have uncontrolled eczema and your GP suspects that diet may be contributing to the eczema
- have eczema that your GP suspects has become infected with the *herpes* virus (eczema herpeticum – see Chapter 3).

concern about treatment, referral to a dermatologist is recommended. Hospital specialists in allergy and problems with the immune system (immunologists) may also get involved in the care of patients with difficult eczema, but they are generally trained to advise on what is triggering the eczema rather than how to treat the condition.

Dermatology nurse specialist
Hospital dermatology departments often have highly trained nurses who can get involved in the care of patients referred to hospital for their eczema. These nurses can demonstrate treatment techniques such as the application of emollients, steroids and bandages, and can help educate and support you in managing your eczema. In some dermatology departments the dermatology

nurse specialists run their own clinics, either in the hospital or in the community (for example, in local GP surgeries). Some nurses can also give treatments on prescription without you needing to see your doctor.

Pharmacist

Your pharmacist can give you general advice about your treatments and make sure you understand how to use them safely. Many eczema treatments can be bought over the counter and pharmacists can provide you with help and information when needed. If you need regular prescriptions it is sensible to try to use the same pharmacist so that they can keep good supplies of your treatment and get to know you better.

Dietician

If your doctor feels that diet is affecting your eczema in any way he or she can refer you to a dietician, either in the community or in your local hospital. Dieticians can ensure that any dietary changes are monitored safely without the risk of nutritional deficiencies.

Clinical psychologist

Psychologists can help selected people with eczema in a number of ways. They can provide counselling and support for emotional and psychological problems arising from the eczema. They can also use behavioural therapy techniques to help break any habit (such as scratching) that may be making the eczema worse. Most clinical psychologists are based in hospitals – referral is done through your doctor.

Basic rules for treating eczema

Although there are many different treatments for eczema, your doctor will usually start you on a mild treatment first and step up to stronger treatments if your skin doesn't improve. Most people with eczema can be treated very effectively with creams and ointments alone. This is called topical treatment; it means that the treatments are put on to the skin rather than being taken by mouth. Many different topical therapies are available, but they can be divided into three broad groups: emollients, topical steroids and topical immunomodulators. Emollients are used as the first line, followed by topical steroids and topical immunomodulators as required. Other treatments, such as bandaging, can be used if your eczema doesn't settle with creams and ointments alone. Tablet treatment and light therapy are reserved for people with more severe eczema.

The general order in which eczema treatments are used is illustrated below. The treatment steps are a guide – remember that everybody's eczema is individual. If your eczema is bad your doctor may start you on a stronger treatment first to get control of the condition, and then step down to weaker treatments as your skin improves. Similarly, some people like to use bandages at an earlier stage in their treatment. Your doctor may also prescribe two or three different treatments for different parts of your body at the same time (for example, emollients for your face and topical steroids plus bandaging for your legs and arms). The number of possibilities is very large, so read on to understand how to make your eczema treatments work for you.

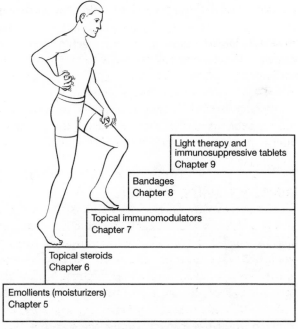

A wide range of treatments are available to help improve
your eczema, ranging from simple emollients to strong tablets.

Chapter 5
Emollients

Emollients are creams, ointments, lotions or gels that keep the skin moist. They are the first and most simple form of treatment you should be given for your eczema, and are used to keep the skin smooth and soft. In eczema the skin tends to dry out very easily. When this occurs then all sorts of things, including infections, irritants and things that you may be allergic to, can get through the skin more easily and make the eczema worse. Emollients provide a protective film over your skin to keep the moisture in and harmful things out. They can also be very soothing and generally make your skin feel more supple and comfortable.

The use of emollients should be encouraged in everyone with atopic eczema, mild or severe. For very mild eczema they may be the only treatment that is needed, although in most people they are used to supplement other treatments such as steroid creams or ointments.

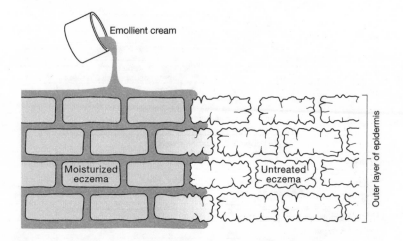

Emollients can help to repair the damaged skin barrier in eczema by replacing the fatty layer of lipid between the skin cells. They act like an artificial mortar, keeping water in the skin and harmful substances out.

Choosing an emollient

Q. There are so many different kinds of moisturizers – how do I know which one is best?

The wide range of emollient preparations can be confusing, but you needn't worry. Everybody with eczema is different and the simple rule is to find an emollient that suits you. This may mean trying several different products until you find an emollient that you find easy and comfortable to use. As a general rule the more greasy the emollient is the more effective it will be at keeping your skin moist. Greasy emollients keep your skin hydrated and protected for longer periods, and are excellent on very dry skin.

Emollient name	Light	Medium	Greasy
Aqueous cream	√		
Aveeno cream®	√		
Aveeno lotion®	√		
Balneum Plus cream®		√	
Cetraben cream®		√	
Dermol 500 lotion®	√		
Dermol cream®		√	
Diprobase cream®		√	
Diprobase ointment®			√
Double base gel®		√	
Dermamist spray®		√	
Epaderm ointment®			√
Emulsifying ointment			√
Eucerin 10% lotion®	√		
Eucerin 10% cream®		√	
E 45 Cream®		√	
Hydrous ointment (oily cream)			√
Hydromol cream®		√	
Hydromol ointment®			√
Liquid & white soft paraffin (50% /50%)			√
Neutrogena dermatological cream®			√
Oilatum cream®		√	
Unguentum M cream®		√	
White soft paraffin			√

Creams are lighter and often easier to use although they need to be applied more often to keep the skin moist. Many people like to use a greasy emollient on their body and a lighter cream on their face, or a greasy emollient at night and a lighter one in the daytime. Most emollients can also be used instead of soap for washing. Your doctor will recommend some suitable emollients to try, and when you have found a preparation that you like it can be put on a regular prescription. You can also buy emollients in your local chemist without a prescription. Most emollients come in big 500 gm tubs or pump dispensers. A list of some of the more common emollients recommended for people with eczema on page 63.

Q. A nurse told me that you can get special emollients to go in the bath. Is this true?
Yes, you can get emollient bath or shower preparations which provide a light greasy layer on the skin after bathing. They are not essential if you are already using a regular emollient at other times, but many children and adults find them easy and pleasant to use. These emollients can make the bath or shower very slippery, so take care and use a non-slip mat. Below are some examples of emollients for the bath or shower.

Emollient bath additives	**Emollient bath additives with added antimicrobial agent**
Aveeno bath oil®	Dermol 600 bath emollient®
Balneum bath oil®	Dermol 200 shower emollient®
Cetraben bath additive®	Emulsiderm liquid emulsion®
Diprobath bath additive®	Oilatum Plus bath additive®
E45 emollient bath oil®	
Hydromol bath additive®	
Oilatum emollient bath additive®	
Oilatum shower emollient®	

How to use emollients

Q. How often should I use my emollient?
Ideally, you should be putting your emollient on at least twice a day, and more frequently if your skin is very dry. One of the best times to put your emollient on is after a warm bath – pat the skin dry with

a soft towel and apply the emollient gently. In the daytime you can use it regularly as often as you want. Emollients are very safe to use anywhere on the body and cannot be overused. You should try to get into the habit of using your emollient every day, even when your eczema is clear as this can reduce the number of flare-ups you get. In babies and young children a layer of emollient on the face before mealtimes can reduce irritation from foods and dribbling. In older children and adults it can be helpful to put emollient on before certain activities such as swimming, going out in cold weather or gardening to protect your skin from irritation. You can keep an extra pot of emollient at school or work for regular use in the daytime. Don't put a thick layer of greasy emollient on immediately before or after applying other treatments such as steroid creams – try to allow at least half an hour to an hour between the two or the emollient may dilute the effect of the steroid.

Q. What is the best way to apply my emollient?
Emollients should be applied gently in the direction of the hairs as they lie on the skin – that is, apply downwards on the arms and legs. Avoid rubbing the skin vigorously in a circular motion as this can aggravate the eczema. Vigorous rubbing of greasy emollients can also cause inflammation of the hair follicles (folliculitis), which appears as tiny red or pus-filled spots around the base of each body hair.

Q. Can I use an emollient instead of soap if I suffer from eczema?
Yes. Many emollients like aqueous cream, Emulsifying ointment® and Epaderm® can be used as soap substitutes for handwashing or cleansing in the bath or shower. Simply rub the emollient into the skin before rinsing off with water. You could also try one of the specially designed bath additives listed above for bathing and showering. In general, ordinary soaps, perfumed bubble baths and shower gels should all be avoided if you have eczema as they can irritate your skin.

Q. Should I be using an emollient with an added antibacterial agent to reduce the chance of my eczema getting infected?
If your eczema is frequently getting infected your doctor may

recommend an emollient containing an antibacterial agent to try to reduce your risk of infections (as listed above). Many people do find these preparations helpful, but the antibacterial additives can occasionally cause skin irritation. Simply using a regular moisturizer (with or without added antibacterials) will prevent your skin from getting dry and cracked and this in itself will reduce the chance of bacteria getting into your skin. Remember, if your eczema often gets weepy and crusty you should see your doctor who can take a swab to test for bacteria, and prescribe a course of antibiotics by mouth if necessary (see Chapter 3).

Common questions about emollients

Q. Can emollients cause any side-effects?

Although emollients are generally very safe, occasionally they may cause some skin irritation and stinging. This usually settles after the first day or two of treatment, but if it doesn't, find another emollient that doesn't sting. Remember that if you have very sore, cracked eczema any cream or ointment is likely to sting until the open sores and cracks heal over. Very rarely people can become allergic to their emollient. This is more likely to occur with creams than ointments, because creams are water-based and contain preservatives. If your skin becomes very red and itchy every time you use a certain emollient discuss this with your doctor as you may need patch-testing to exclude an allergy to the cream (see Chapter 11).

Q. I can't seem to find an emollient to suit my child. I've tried several different products but her eczema is really bad and she always cries and screams every time I try and put them on. What do you suggest?

It is unlikely that there is a problem with the emollients that you've tried, as it would be unusual to react to many different preparations. It sounds like your child simply doesn't like having things applied to her skin at the moment. The most common reason is that the eczema is sore and inflamed, and this should settle within a few days if the skin is treated effectively with a topical steroid or other active treatment. However, some children simply don't like having creams and ointments put on, even when their skin isn't sore. This can be a challenging problem for parents but there are various ways of building up a child's confidence and making emollient time a fun activity rather than a battle. Try pretending to apply the emollient to your child's doll or favourite plastic toy before you treat her. Encourage her to get involved and let her help put the emollient on. Find a product that she likes the feel and smell of – try a jelly-like preparation such as Doublebase®, or let her decorate a pump dispenser of Diprobase® or tub of Epaderm®, for example. If your child still refuses to let you use emollients discuss the problem with your doctor or nurse.

Q. My doctor gave me aqueous cream as a moisturizer for my child, but his skin gets very red and itchy every time I use it. Is he allergic to aqueous cream?

A recent study showed that over half of children prescribed aqueous cream actually developed stinging, itching, redness or burning after application of the product. These side-effects are usually caused by irritation rather than true contact allergy, and may vary between different aqueous cream preparations because different manufacturers often use different preservatives. Aqueous cream was originally designed to be used as a wash product rather than a leave-on emollient, and many children find they can use it as a soap substitute with no problems, even if it irritates them when left on the skin. The simple message is to change to a different emollient and find one that your child likes. If your child seems to be reacting to specific emollients see your doctor to discuss whether he needs patch-testing (see Chapter 8).

Using emollients in different types of eczema

Q. My baby has a few small patches of pink scaly eczema on his face and body. What should I use to moisturize his skin?

It sounds like your baby's eczema is very mild. If he isn't scratch-ing and don't seem troubled by his skin there is no reason to use a steroid cream at the moment. A simple light or moderately greasy emollient (see table on page 63) will help – use it two or three times a day and after bathing to keep the skin smooth and reduce the chance of the eczema progressing. Very greasy emollients such as liquid paraffin and white soft paraffin aren't usually needed in very young babies, and occasionally clog the skin or cause a mild folliculitis in tiny infants. Remember to avoid products that may irritate and dry your baby's skin such as soaps, detergents, wool and extremes of temperature.

Q. My baby has bad cradle cap. Would an emollient help?
Yes. Thick scalp scales will usually lift off easily with gentle combing if you apply a greasy emollient (such as Epaderm®) several times a day, followed by washing with a simple baby shampoo. Alternatively, warm olive oil can be massaged into the scalp and left on for an hour before combing. Tar-based shampoos such as Capasal® can sometimes be useful in small amounts but should be stopped if they irritate the skin. If the scale is stuck on don't try to pick it off as you may leave your baby's skin sore and red. Be gentle and don't scrub the scalp or you may aggravate the condition. If the scale is very thick see your health visitor or doctor before trying to treat the scalp yourself.

Q. My teenage son has very thick dry eczema on the legs and arms. He always uses a light moisturizer from over the counter but it sinks in straight away and the skin stays looking dry and leathery. Any suggestions?
Thick lichenified eczema responds best to greasy emollients such as Hydromol ointment or 50/50 liquid paraffin/white soft paraffin. If your son is not keen to use greasy emollients in the daytime try to encourage him to use them at night, with a less greasy product in the daytime (see table on page 63). Bandaging with wet wraps over a greasy emollient at night can be very useful to treat this type of eczema (see Chapter 8).

Q. I am a mother of two young children and have suffered from hand eczema for the last 12 months. What is the best emollient to use?
There are no hard-and-fast rules – it depends which emollient you find easiest to use. You need to get in the habit of using an emollient instead of soap every time you wash your hands as well as a regular emollient throughout the day. A preparation that works as a soap-substitute as well as a leave-on emollient may be

the best, for example, Epaderm®, Diprobase®, or emulsifying ointment. Make sure you avoid direct contact with detergents, soaps and cleaning agents, and wear gloves with cotton liners when washing up. Try not to wear your gloves for long periods at a time, and avoid exposure to very hot water when washing up – too much heat will make your hands sweaty in your gloves and exacerbate your eczema. If you can, get a dishwasher. Make sure you remove all your rings before doing any housework, because water and irritants can collect under the rings and trigger new areas of eczema. When preparing food avoid handling acidic fruits, chillies, onions or garlic with bare hands as these can all irritate the skin.

If these simple measures fail to clear your skin see your doctor, who can prescribe a stronger treatment (for example, a topical steroid) or arrange further investigations as necessary.

Q. My mother has recently gone into a nursing home and her legs have become very dry and cracked. Would she benefit from an emollient?

Asteatotic eczema (see Chapter 1) is very common in the elderly, especially during the winter months. It can be caused by bathing too often in hot soapy water or as a result of living in an environment with low humidity and high temperature. Check which products are being used to bathe your mother and ensure she is not sitting by direct heat. A regular emollient will certainly help the problem, and is probably all that is needed if her skin is dry rather than red and inflamed. A moderately greasy or very greasy emollient such as Cetraben® or Epaderm® is best as it won't need to be applied as frequently as lighter products. The emollient can also be used in the shower or bath, providing a non-slip mat is used. Advise the staff and carers in the nursing home to avoid using bubble baths, soaps, talcum powder and other perfumed products which may all irritate your mother's skin.

Chapter 6
Topical steroids

Topical steroids (also called corticosteroids) have formed the main treatment for people with eczema over the last fifty years. Steroids are naturally occurring hormones that are produced by the body in small amounts for normal growth and development. A number of synthetic steroids have been developed over the years to treat people with skin conditions such as eczema and psoriasis. When applied to the skin topical steroids are very effective at reducing skin inflammation, controlling symptoms and restoring one's quality of life. The widespread use of topical steroids over many years has provided doctors and nurses with plenty of experience in how they can be used effectively without causing side-effects. Without a doubt when topical steroids are used properly they are extremely safe and provide one of the most valuable treatments currently available for people with eczema.

Topical steroid strengths
In the UK topical steroids come in four strengths (see Table 1):

- mild (or weak)
- moderately potent (or moderately strong)
- potent (strong)
- very potent (very strong).

There is an enormous difference in strength (and potential side-effects) between steroids in these four categories. A very potent steroid such as Dermovate® is over a thousand times as strong as a mild steroid such as hydrocortisone. The basic principle is to use the mildest steroid that will control your eczema, as stronger preparations have a higher risk of side-effects if not used correctly. This means that your doctor will usually start with a mild preparation and step up to a moderately potent or potent preparation if your eczema is not responding. If your eczema is bad it is sometimes better to start with a potent preparation to get quick control, and then step down gradually to a moderate or weak preparation as your eczema clears. One of the best ways to use topical steroids is in short bursts, stopping when the eczema clears and restarting when it flares up again. Using steroids in this way reduces the chances of side-effects and also prevents the effectiveness of the steroid from wearing off over time (called tachyphylaxis), which can occur with continuous daily use.

Understanding topical steroids

Q. How do topical steroids work in eczema?
Topical steroids reduce inflammation in the skin. The way in which they do this is very complicated but basically the steroids temporarily alter the function of some of the immune cells, blood vessels and chemicals in the skin. This dampens down the abnormal reactions occurring in eczema and helps the skin to clear.

Q. Are steroid creams and ointments dangerous?
No, not at all if used sensibly. Unfortunately, when steroid creams were first introduced widely in the 1960s they were so effective that many people used potent preparations inappropriately for months or years without stopping, and this resulted in adverse side-effects. The stronger the steroid is the more potential it has to cause side-effects. The most common side-effect of topical steroids is thinning of the skin. The skin becomes wrinkly and papery with tiny blood vessels (called telangiectasia) visible. With more prolonged use, strong steroids can sometimes cause stretch marks like women can get in pregnancy (called striae). Although mild skin thinning can be reversible if the steroid is stopped, if stretch marks develop they are usually permanent. It must be stressed that skin damage from steroid creams and ointments is now extremely uncommon and should not occur if the treatments are used properly. Unfortunately, because of the problems seen many years ago some people remain frightened of topical steroids and under-use their creams and ointments – this stops them taking full control of their eczema. If topical steroids are used properly the potential for damage is very small compared with the potential damage of

leaving your eczema untreated, which can make life a misery. If you or your GP has any concerns about the side-effects of topical steroids, arrange to be referred to your local dermatologist to discuss your concerns further.

Q. Will steroid creams affect the growth and development of my child?

No, this is extremely unlikely. Steroid creams and ointments should not be confused with steroid tablets or anabolic steroids taken by athletes, which can affect growth and development. This is because steroid tablets are absorbed into your bloodstream and can reduce your body's production of natural steroids. The standard amounts of topical steroid used for eczema treatment will not be absorbed through the skin in sufficient amounts to have any effect on growth and development, or affect your child's ability to fight infections. Significant absorption of steroid cream is a potential problem only if strong topical steroids are used on large areas of the body for long periods of time, especially under bandages or in very young children. The use of strong topical steroids in this way is not recommended except under the close supervision of a dermatologist in a hospital setting who would ensure that there was no long-term risk to your child.

Q. Do topical steroids have any other side-effects?

Yes, they do but these are not common. When used on the face and upper body topical steroids can occasionally cause acne, or a spotty rash around the mouth called perioral dermatitis. Steroids can sometimes cause small inflamed spots around the hair follicles (called folliculitis). If topical steroids are used for long periods they can cause a temporary mild increase in fine-hair growth in the treated skin, although this is rare. Mild and temporary decreases in skin pigment are also occasionally seen, although it is much more common for the eczema itself to cause skin pigment changes (see below).

Q I have black skin. Will topical steroids leave me with pale patches on my skin?

This is unlikely. Very occasionally steroid creams can cause some mild temporary skin lightening but this should return to normal after you stop using them. You are more likely to develop discolouration of your skin if you leave your eczema untreated. This is because skin inflammation can affect the distribution of pigment in your skin. If you have very inflamed eczema it is common to be left with either pale or dark patches of skin which can last for several months even after the eczema has cleared. Doctors call this appearance post-inflammatory hypopigmentation (skin lightening) or hyperpigmentation (skin darkening). Similar pigment changes can also occur after other inflammatory skin conditions such as psoriasis. Post-inflammatory hypo- or hyperpigmentation can affect anyone regardless of their underlying skin colour, although the changes are usually more obvious in Asian or Afro-Caribbean skin.

Q. Can I become allergic to my steroid creams?

Yes, you can, but this is very uncommon. It is much more common for steroid creams and ointments to simply irritate or sting your skin for a few minutes when they are first put on, especially if your eczema is very inflamed and red. This usually settles as your eczema improves.

True topical steroid allergy is rare. If it occurs it causes an allergic contact dermatitis (see Chapter 1). The symptoms appear as a worsening of your eczema, often a few hours or even days after putting the steroid on to your skin. The most common ingredients in steroid creams and ointments that people become allergic to are:

- **preservatives in the steroid**: steroid creams are more likely to cause an allergy than ointments because they contain preservatives, whereas ointments generally don't
- **antibiotics in the steroid**: some topical steroids contain antibiotics which can occasionally cause a contact allergy. Some antibiotics such as neomycin are more likely to cause allergy than others – look at the ingredients in the small print on your tube of steroid to find out what is in it
- **the steroid itself**: you can become allergic to the steroid chemical itself in either steroid creams or ointments, but this is rare.

If you think that your eczema is definitely getting worse every time you use your topical steroid you should discuss this with your doctor, who can refer you to the hospital for patch-testing if necessary (see Chapter 11).

Q. Can I buy steroid creams and ointments over the counter without a prescription from my doctor?

Yes, you can. In the UK two types of topical steroid can be bought from your local pharmacist without a prescription – hydrocortisone (0.1 per cent, 0.5 per cent and 1 per cent – all mild) and Eumovate® (moderately potent). You can buy both of these preparations to treat eczema, contact dermatitis and insect bites. However, pharmacists are not allowed to advise you to use these topical steroids on your face or genital region, on broken or infected skin or in children under the age of ten. It is recommended that this kind of use should be supervised by a doctor.

Q. Will steroid creams make me grow out of my eczema more slowly?

There is no evidence that topical steroids or any other treatments change the underlying natural course of skin disease – that is, they don't seem to make people grow out of their eczema any slower or any quicker.

Q. What is the point of using steroid creams when they aren't getting to the cause of my eczema?

You are right that topical steroids will only suppress your eczema and not cure it. For some types of eczema, such as contact eczema, you may be able to 'cure' your eczema by avoiding contact with the substances causing the problem. However, for many common types of eczema, including atopic eczema, the causes are much more complicated and sadly there isn't yet a cure. Some of the causes of atopic eczema (such as the genes you are born with) simply cannot be changed, and many of the common environmental triggers such as house dust mite are impossible to avoid completely without making life extremely difficult. Understandably, many people find this frustrating because they feel that their treatments aren't getting to the root of the problem. Despite this, treatments such as topical steroids do offer the best solution for clearing your skin, overcoming your symptoms and helping you get on with your life.

Q. How long will I need to use my topical steroids for?

You will need to use all your treatments on and off for as long as your eczema lasts. Almost three-quarters of children grow out of their eczema by early teenage years. However, a few people continue to have symptoms throughout their adult life and may need to use topical steroids on and off for many years.

How to use your topical steroids

Q. How many times a day should I use my steroid ointment?

You should never use your steroid cream or ointment more than twice a day – this will not make it more effective and may increase the risk of side-effects. Most topical steroid preparations have traditionally been used twice daily. However, there is not much research evidence that twice-daily treatment is any better than once-daily treatment. Therefore it is sensible to try once-daily treatment first, and move up to twice daily if this fails. Some topical steroids such as Elocon® are specifically marketed for once-daily use only.

Q. How much steroid cream or ointment do I need to use?

You will need a thin layer of topical steroid over any areas of skin where the eczema is active (red and itchy). Do not use your topical steroid as an emollient just to keep your skin moisturized. If your skin is not itchy or red, and you have no symptoms, do not put it on – just use your emollient. The fingertip rule is a useful guide to how much steroid you should be using. Squeeze a length of steroid (cream or ointment) from your tube on to the tip of an adult index finger, starting at the tip of the finger and stopping at the first finger crease you come to. This small length of steroid (approximately 2 cm) is one fingertip unit, and should be enough to cover an area of skin twice the size of a flat adult hand. One fingertip unit weighs approximately 0.5 gm (a standard tube of steroid contains 30 gm). Your doctor or nurse may ask you to bring your tubes of steroid to your appointments. This is so they can get an idea of how much steroid you are using and advise you if they feel you are over- or under-using your steroid.

Q. When is the best time to put my steroid ointment on?

If you are using a once-daily topical steroid one of the best times to put it on is in the evening after a warm bath. A twice-daily steroid can be put on after a shower in the morning, and in the evening before bedtime. Although this regime suits most people there are no hard-and-fast rules. As long as you are finding time to get the treatment on just find a time that fits in best with your lifestyle. It is a good idea to put your topical steroid on an hour or more before bedtime to give it time to sink into the skin. This is especially important if you are using a potent steroid, because it will avoid transferring it to other parts of your body in your sleep. If you are using steroid creams to treat your child's hand eczema, a pair of cotton gloves can be useful at night time to prevent your child rubbing it on to his or her face while sleeping. You can use as much emollient as you want, but try to leave a gap of at least half an hour to an hour between applying your topical steroid and your emollient – this will avoid diluting the steroid and reducing its effectiveness.

Q. Are steroid ointments better than creams?

Ointments are generally better for people with eczema for two reasons. First, they are greasier so they have a better moisturizing effect on dry skin and this may help the steroid work more effectively. Second, ointments don't contain preservatives, whereas creams do. Very occasionally preservatives can cause skin irritation or contact allergy (see Chapter 11). However, many people prefer a cream on the face as it is more cosmetically acceptable.

Q. It says on the information leaflet that my steroid cream shouldn't be used on broken skin. Does this mean I can't use it if my eczema is weepy and cracked?

Under the supervision of your doctor it is perfectly all right to use a topical steroid on your eczema even when the skin is broken and inflamed. The skin is often broken and cracked if you have bad eczema, and topical steroids are one of the best ways of helping the skin to return to normal. The advice on your information leaflet is provided because topical steroids are more easily absorbed through broken skin, but as long as they are used for short bursts under the supervision of your doctor and stopped when the skin returns to normal they are absolutely safe.

Q. My eczema has cleared completely with a short burst of Betnovate®. If I put some Betnovate® on every now and then will it help to stop my eczema from coming back?

Doctors usually recommend that you stop your steroid as soon as your eczema clears and start it again only when it starts to come back. However, some people find that their eczema flares up very quickly as soon as they stop the steroid. So can steroid creams be used to *prevent* the eczema from flaring up again, instead of waiting for the flare-up to occur? Some recent research trials have looked at this question in more detail. These trials suggest that in adults with moderate to severe eczema the use of a potent topical steroid on two consecutive days a week (for example, at weekends only) can reduce the risk of flare-ups without evidence of side-effects such as skin thinning. In these trials the potent steroid was applied to the healed areas where the eczema usually occurred as well as to any new patches of eczema. Although these trials have been helpful there is still not enough evidence to suggest that preventative treatment in this way is suitable for people with milder eczema, or for children with eczema. If you repeatedly get patches of eczema flaring up in the same sites, discuss with your doctor whether weekend topical steroid treatment may be helpful.

Q. My GP has given me a steroid cream with an antibacterial agent in it. Is this better for my eczema than a tube of plain steroid?

No, for regular treatment of your eczema there is no good evidence that a steroid with an antibacterial agent (see Table 2 on page 81) is any better than a plain steroid cream. Some people find a two-week course of a steroid/antibiotic cream helps if their eczema becomes red and inflamed, and this may be because there is some mild bacterial infection in the eczema. However, you should not continue to use the steroid/antibiotic cream for more than two weeks except in special circumstances under your doctor's guidance. This is because continued use can cause the bacteria on your skin to become resistant to the antibiotic, thus decreasing its effectiveness. Very occasionally you can also develop an allergy to the antibiotic. Plain steroids alone will reduce the number of bacteria on your skin very effectively simply by restoring the damaged skin to normal. If your eczema becomes very infected (see Chapter 3) a short course of antibiotics by mouth is usually much more effective than a steroid/antibiotic cream.

Q. Are topical steroids with added antifungal ingredients helpful for atopic eczema?
Mild topical steroids with antifungal action (listed in Table 2 on page 81) are mainly used to treat people with seborrhoeic eczema. Some patients with other types of eczema find a combined steroid/anti-fungal/antibacterial cream such as Trimovate® (moderately potent) very useful for treating eczema in warm moist areas such as the genitals. In these areas the eczema is prone to getting infected with both bacteria and a yeast (type of fungus) called *candida*.

Getting to grips with using different strengths of topical steroids

Q. I always come away from the doctor's surgery with a bag of different creams and ointments. By the time I get home I can't always remember what to use where and when. I don't like to keep bothering the doctor but I really do get confused.
There are so many different topical steroid and emollient prepara-tions that treatment really can get quite confusing. Ask your doctor and nurse to write down a treatment plan for you to follow. Ideally you should ask them to show you how to use the creams as well. If you see a hospital specialist ask him or her to send you a typed copy of the letter that is sent to your GP – this should detail all your treatments. A written record is one of the best ways of getting to grips with your treatments – it will help you know and remember the strengths of your topical steroids and when to use them. Once you have mastered this you can safely and effectively get straight on top of any flare-ups before they get out of control. Also, if you have ongoing chronic eczema it helps to try to see the same doctor or nurse each time so that you both get to know each other and there is continuity in your care.

Q. I find it hard to remember the names and strengths of all the different steroid creams I have been given in the past. Is it important to know the difference?

It is very important to know the strength of any topical steroids that you are using. This is because when your eczema is bad you will need a stronger topical steroid than when your eczema is under control. Strong steroid ointments should also be avoided on parts of the body with delicate skin (see below).To be in control of eczema most people find that they need two or three different strengths of topical steroid at home so that they can alter their treatment depending on how bad the eczema is and which part of the body is affected (see below).

Q. How can I find out how strong my topical steroids are? The strength isn't mentioned on the tube.

You can check the strength of any topical steroids you are given in the two tables on the following pages – they list the preparations currently available in the UK and their potency. Table 1 shows the different topical steroid preparations which you might be prescribed, and Table 2 shows the topical steroids that contain added ingredients to fight bacteria or fungi (antimicrobial agents). In both tables the percentage (%) figure given after the steroid name in the second column refers to the dilution of the steroid, and not the strength. This percentage figure can be misleading because a diluted potent steroid can still be stronger than a less-diluted mild steroid. The last column (headed 'Strength') in both tables indicates the strength of the steroids.

There are many different topical steroid preparations available in the UK, and it is easy to get confused, as you can end up with several different tubes of steroid at home, prescribed by different doctors over the years.

Remember that every time your doctor or nurse prescribes you a topical steroid they should tell you how strong it is. Ask them to write down the strengths of all your steroid ointments on a treatment plan if you are at all unsure. Try to stick to one or two different topical steroids that you can become familiar with to avoid any confusion, and remember to take the tubes with you each time you visit your doctor or nurse.

Table 1 Plain topical steroids

Trade name *(this is the name chosen by the manufacturer – it is in big print on the tube)*	Generic name *(this is the official name of the steroid – it is usually written in smaller print on the tube)*	Strength *(Potency)*
Hydrocortisone 0.5%	hydrocortisone 0.5%, 1%	mild
Dioderm®	hydrocortisone 0.1%	mild
Efcortelan®	hydrocortisone 0.5%, 1%, 2.5%	mild
Mildison®	hydrocortisone 1%	mild
Synalar 1 in 10®	fluocinolone acetonide 0.0025%	mild
Modrasone®	alclometasone dipropionate 0.05%	moderate
Betnovate-RD®	betamethasone valerate 0.025%	moderate
Eumovate®	clobetasone butyrate 0.05%	moderate
Haelan®	fludroxycortide 0.0125%	moderate
Synalar 1 in 4®	fluocinolone acetonide 0.00625%	moderate
Diprosone®	betamethasone dipropionate 0.05%	potent
Elocon®	mometasone furoate 0.1%	potent
Metosyn®	fluocinonide 0.05%	potent
Cutivate®	fluticasone propionate 0.05%/0.005%	potent
Stiedex lotion®	desoximetasone 0.25%	potent
Locoid®	hydrocortisone butyrate 0.1%	potent
Nerisone®	diflucortolone valerate 0.1%	potent
Synalar®	fluocinolone acetonide 0.025%	potent
Propaderm®	beclometasone dipropionate 0.025%	potent
Betnovate®	betamethasone valerate 0.1%	potent
Dermovate®	clobetasol propionate 0.05%	very potent
Halciderm topical®	halcinonide 0.1%	very potent
Nerisone Forte®	diflucortolone valerate 0.3%	very potent

Table 2 Topical steroids with added antimicrobial effects

Sometimes used for short bursts if infection with bacteria or fungi is suspected.

Trade name	Generic name	Main antimicrobial	Added antimicrobial effect	Strength
Canesten HC®	hydrocortisone 1%	antifungal	clotrimazole	mild
Daktacort®	hydrocortisone 1%	antifungal	miconazole nitrate	mild
Econacort®	hydrocortisone 1%	antifungal	econazole nitrate	mild
Fucidin H®	hydrocortisone 1%	antibacterial	fusidic acid	mild
Nystaform HC®	hydrocortisone 0.5%	antifungal	nystatin	mild
		antibacterial	chlorhexidine hydrochloride	mild
Timodine®	hydrocortisone 0.5%	antibacterial	benzalkonium chloride	mild
		antifungal	nystatin	mild
Vioform-Hydrocortisone®	hydrocortisone 1%	antibacterial	clioquinol	mild
Trimovate®	clobetasone butyrate 0.05%	antibacterial	oxytetracycline	moderate
		antifungal	nystatin	moderate
Aureocort®	triamcinolone acetonide 0.1%	antibacterial	chlortetracycline hydrochloride	potent
Betnovate-C®	betamethasone valerate 0.1%	antibacterial	clioquinol	potent
Betnovate-N®	betamethasone valerate 0.1%	antibacterial	neomycin sulphate	potent
Fucibet®	betamethasone valerate 0.1%	antibacterial	fusidic acid	potent
Locoid C®	hydrocortisone butyrate 0.1%	antibacterial	chlorquinaldol	potent
Lotriderm®	betamethasone dipropionate 0.064%	antifungal	clotrimazole	potent
Synalar C®	fluocinolone acetonide 0.025%	antibacterial	clioquinol	potent
Synalar N®	fluocinolone acetonide 0.025%	antifungal	neomycin sulphate	potent
Tri-Adcortyl®	triamcinolone acetonide 0.1%	antibacterial	neomycin gramicidin	potent
		antifungal	nystatin	potent
Dermovate-NN®	clobetasol propionate 0.05%	antibacterial	neomycin	v. potent
		antifungal	nystatin	v. potent

Q. Why has my doctor given me one steroid cream for the body and a different one for the face?

You have been given different creams because the skin on the face is much more delicate than that on the body, and so steroid creams are more easily absorbed and have more potential to cause side-effects. In general, potent or very potent topical steroids should not be used for eczema on the face (except in very special circumstances under the supervision of a dermatologist) as there is a risk of causing skin thinning and the appearance of visible tiny blood vessels (telangiectasia). If emollient treatment alone is not controlling your facial eczema your doctor may prescribe a weak or moderately potent steroid cream which should be used for a few days at a time as directed, avoiding the very delicate skin around the eyes as much as possible. Fortunately, eczema on the face rarely becomes thick and chronic, and usually clears well with a few days of using 1 per cent hydrocortisone cream.

On the body the skin is thicker and potent topical steroids can be used safely in short bursts under your doctor's supervision. The only exception is in the skin creases (sometimes called flexures) such as the neck, under the arms, in front of the elbows, behind the knees and in the groins or nappy area. Like the face these areas have thinner and more delicate skin and in general only weak or moderately potent topical steroids should be used. Occasionally, stronger steroids are needed (under your doctor's supervision), especially for longstanding thick eczema behind the knees or around the elbows. However, if you need to use potent topical steroids in the skin creases on a regular basis you should ideally be supervised by a dermatologist.

Q. Which steroid creams can be used around the eyes?

The skin around the eyes is very delicate and topical steroids should be avoided in this area as much as possible. If you get eczema on your eyelids or around your eyes try a simple emollient cream first. If this fails, a few days of using 1 per cent hydrocortisone is usually sufficient (under your doctor's supervision), but it should not be continued for long periods. If stronger steroids are used around the eyes (or occasionally if weak steroids are used for long periods), the pressure inside the eye may increase (glaucoma), and very occasionally cataracts can develop which interfere with vision. Protopic® and Elidel® (see Chapter 7) are useful alternatives to topical steroids if you are getting lots of eczema around your eyes – discuss this with your doctor.

Q. My child has stubborn patches of eczema on the hands and feet which have not cleared with hydrocortisone. What should I use?

The skin on the palms of the hands and soles of the feet is very thick, and steroid creams do not get absorbed very easily through thick skin. Weak topical steroids often don't work very well on these areas, and if your child's eczema has not cleared with a mild or moderately potent steroid such as hydrocortisone or Eumovate®, your doctor may recommend a short burst of a potent steroid. Remember that the skin on the backs of the hands and the tops of the feet is much thinner than the palms and soles so topical steroids should be used for shorter periods in these areas.

Q. Should my six-month-old baby be using weaker topical steroids than my nine-year-old child?

As a general rule young children are more susceptible to the potential side-effects of steroid creams and ointments than older children and adults, for two reasons. First, a baby's skin is thinner and more delicate. Second, babies and young children have a large surface area of skin compared to their body size – this means that they can potentially absorb more steroid cream for their body weight compared with an older child or adult.

Fortunately, most babies and young infants with eczema respond well to intermittent treatment with a weak steroid such as 1 per cent hydrocortisone, which is extremely safe. Infants and preschool children whose eczema fails to improve with hydrocortisone can be treated with short bursts of a moderately potent steroid such as Eumovate ointment® under a doctor's supervision. If their eczema is still not controlled, they should be referred to a skin specialist, who can ensure that all the treatments are being used properly. The skin specialist can supervise short bursts of a potent steroid if indicated, and will refer you back to your GP's care once your child's eczema is under control using a safe treatment regime.

School children should also start off using a weak or moderately potent topical steroid, but may need intermittent short bursts (say, three days) of a potent topical steroid on the body, legs or arms if the eczema doesn't clear, again under a doctor's supervision. If a school-age child needs to use potent topical steroids for longer bursts on a regular basis, they should usually be reviewed by a skin specialist. Many children do need potent topical steroids for longer bursts but it is always best to ensure that other aspects of their treatment are optimal first. Very potent topical steroids such as Dermovate® are only used in children in very exceptional circumstances and should be supervised by a skin specialist.

Q. I have had eczema all my life. What strengths of steroid are safe for me to use as an adult?

There are no hard-and-fast rules to say when different strengths of topical steroids can be used safely as it will depend on the site, type and severity of your eczema. Your doctor will be able to guide you, based on the appearance of your skin and how much your eczema is bothering you. Most adults can control their eczema with one-to-two-week bursts of a mild, moderately potent or potent topical steroid, with shorter bursts if the eczema clears more quickly. As discussed above you should stick to a mild or moderately potent topical steroid to treat your face and skin creases, but you may need a potent preparation for your legs, arms and body. Very potent steroids such as Dermovate® are rarely needed, but can be useful for a few days at a time under your doctor's supervision to treat very thick stubborn patches of eczema (not on the face). Discuss these options with your doctor, who will advise you on the best treatment for you as an individual.

Q. Is 1 per cent hydrocortisone stronger than 0.1 per cent Betnovate?

No, this is a very common mistake that people make. Unfortunately, the percentage strengths on the tubes can be very confusing as they do not relate to the potency of the topical steroid (as illustrated in Table 1 on page 80). All forms of hydrocortisone are classified as *mild* steroids, including the 0.1 per cent,

0.5 per cent and 1 per cent preparations. Betnovate® (cream, ointment, lotion or scalp application) is a *potent* steroid. This means that all standard preparations of Betnovate® are stronger than hydrocortisone. A diluted form of Betnovate is available called Betnovate-RD® – this is classified as a *moderately potent steroid* because it contains standard-strength Betnovate which has been diluted four times. Betnovate-RD® is still stronger than hydrocortisone. Remember – if you are in any doubt about how strong your topical steroid is, ask your doctor, nurse or pharmacist who will be more than happy to answer your questions.

Q. My GP has given me Locoid ointment® and told me that it is a potent steroid. In small letters on the tube it says that it contains hydrocortisone butyrate so is it really a mild steroid after all?

No, your GP is right. If you stick to reading the main name on your steroid tube (trade name) which will be written in big letters you will not get confused. Locoid® is made from hydrocortisone butyrate which is a *potent* steroid. Hydrocortisone butyrate is not the same as hydrocortisone, which is a mild steroid.

Q. Since my teenage years I have noticed that my eczema has become very thick and dry, especially on my arms and legs. What sort of topical steroid is best for this type of eczema?

Your skin becomes thickened in response to chronic scratching over long periods of time – doctors call this 'lichenification'. If you look closely at normal skin you will see a pattern of tiny lines called skin markings. In longstanding areas of eczema these skin markings become much more visible – this is a sign that the skin has become thickened or lichenified. Lichenification is most often seen around the joints, especially on the legs and arms. It is more common in adults who have had eczema for years, but can also develop in children, especially if the eczema has not been well controlled. When lichenification occurs, steroid creams and ointments can't get into thick scaly skin as easily as they can into early thin patches of eczema. This means that short bursts of potent topical steroids are often required (under a doctor's supervision), although the steroid should be stopped when the skin returns to normal texture. If your skin remains thick and dry after a burst of steroid but the itching has settled, try using just your emollient until it returns to normal. Sometimes lichenified areas can take several weeks to completely return to normal skin texture even after your symptoms have settled.

Q. Should I use long bursts of a weak steroid or shorter bursts of a strong steroid to clear my child's eczema?

If your child's eczema is clearing with either regime it probably doesn't matter too much whether you choose to stick to a weak steroid or use a slightly stronger steroid for a shorter burst. Stronger steroids will usually bring the eczema under control more quickly and therefore don't need to be used for as long. However, some people prefer to stick to a weaker preparation that can be safely used on both the face and body to keep things simple.

A recent study in Nottingham has shown that in children aged between one and fifteen years with mild to moderate eczema, three-day bursts of a potent steroid ointment (Betnovate®) were as effective as seven-day bursts of a mild steroid ointment (1 per cent hydrocortisone) for treating eczema flare-ups. Both regimes were safe and equally effective overall. No evidence of skin thinning or other important side-effects was seen with either treatment.

Q. I keep getting bad eczema on my scalp. It is very scaly and the itch is driving me mad. Which steroid preparations can be used on this area?

It is very common to get eczema on the scalp, although your doctor should examine you to make sure there is no other cause for your itching such as ringworm infection or head lice (see Chapter 1). A variety of different scalp steroid preparations are available – these are all potent or very potent steroids as weaker steroids don't work well on thick scalp skin. It is important that the product is applied only to the scalp and not allowed to drip down on to the face or neck, where it may cause side-effects. Such steroids are available in the form of lotions, gels and mousses, so find a preparation that suits your lifestyle. Most people prefer to apply their scalp product at night as it can make the hair look greasy. It can be washed off in the morning with a simple non-perfumed shampoo. Some steroid scalp preparations contain alcohol, which can sting. If your eczema is very inflamed try a non-alcoholic-based product such as Synalar gel®.

As with steroid treatment on other parts of the body, you should use your steroid scalp application for intermittent bursts when you need it rather than every day. You may need to treat your scalp every night for a week or two to bring the eczema under control, followed by intermittent treatment as required. Many people need to use their scalp treatment only once a week or less to keep their eczema under control.

Examples of steroid scalp applications include:

- Betnovate scalp application® (potent)
- Bettamousse foam® (potent)
- Locoid scalp lotion® (potent)
- Synalar gel® (potent)
- Dermovate scalp application® (very potent).

Q. My son keeps getting tiny spots around the hairs on his legs whenever he uses his Betnovate. Is it too strong for him?

It sounds like your son is getting folliculitis (inflammation in the hair follicles). This is a common problem and can be caused by topical steroids, although it is not necessarily because his topical steroid is too strong for him (discuss this with your doctor). Folliculitis can also be caused by overuse of thick greasy emollients, or by incorrect technique in putting the topical steroids or emollients on to the skin. Make sure he is applying his topical steroids and emollients in a thin layer in the direction of the hair growth on the skin rather than rubbing the ointment in using a circular or up-and-down motion. If he is using a very greasy emollient such as liquid paraffin/white soft paraffin or Epaderm®, try swapping to a lighter emollient such as Diprobase®, Cetraben® or aqueous cream. An emollient containing an antiseptic such as Dermol 500® or an antibacterial bath additive may also help. If the problem persists try swapping to a less potent steroid such as Eumovate®, depending on the severity of his eczema and after discussion with your doctor.

Q. My skin gets red and scaly around the sides of my nose, in my eyebrows and on my scalp. My GP has given me a mild steroid/antifungal cream. Is this safe on the face?

It sounds like you are suffering from seborrhoeic eczema (see Chapter 1). This type of eczema can be associated with an overgrowth of a common yeast (type of fungus) on the skin. This yeast (called *malassezia furfur*) lives on many people's skin and causes no problems, but people with seborrhoeic eczema can react to the yeast and develop skin inflammation. If antifungal creams are used regularly the yeast levels on the skin can be kept low enough not to cause a problem. A plain antifungal cream such as Nizoral® (ketoconazole 2 per cent cream) may be sufficient to treat your eczema, although many people find that a combined steroid/antifungal cream is more effective as the topical steroid helps to reduce the inflammation. If you are using a topical steroid/antifungal try to stick to a mild preparation containing hydrocortisone such as Daktacort® and avoid the area around the eyes. Use the treatment only when the skin is red and scaly, for two- or three-week bursts if possible – this is very unlikely to cause any side-effects. If you need to use your steroid continuously for weeks or months, have a chat with your doctor about alternative treatments. On the scalp a plain antifungal shampoo such as Nizoral shampoo® may keep on top of your dandruff, although a potent topical steroid scalp preparation may be needed for short bursts (see above).

Q. My ten-week-old baby has red shiny skin in his groins, under his arms and around his neck. My doctor has told me it is seborrhoeic eczema and has prescribed hydrocortisone cream but is this safe to use on a baby?

If simple emollients have not helped, your baby would probably benefit from a short course of a mild topical steroid such as hydrocortisone. Doctors do have to be careful with topical steroids in very young children as their skin is thin and delicate, especially in the skin creases. This means that steroid creams should be used only for short periods of time under a doctor's supervision. Fortunately, your baby's skin will probably clear up with a few days of topical hydrocortisone, and you can then continue with just emollients. His seborrhoeic eczema will have a tendency to come and go for the first few months of life and may need further short courses of hydrocortisone. This is perfectly safe if you need the treatment only for intermittent bursts and your doctor is keeping an eye on how much topical steroid you are using each month. The link between skin yeasts and seborrhoeic eczema is less clear in children than in adults, and combined topical steroid/antifungal preparations are generally less helpful than they are for adults with seborrhoeic eczema.

If the nappy area is affected it is important to keep the skin very clean and dry to prevent infection. Change nappies frequently or as soon as they become wet or dirty, and use an emollient to protect the skin after every nappy change.

Q. I keep getting tiny blisters along the sides of my fingers which my doctor tells me is pompholyx eczema. Hydrocortisone ointment hasn't worked so what do you suggest?

Moderate or potent topical steroids are usually required for several days to settle down an acute episode of pompholyx. Steroid creams are often easier to use than greasy ointments on wet, weeping skin. Cotton gloves and socks can also be worn on top of your topical steroid under your doctor's supervision – this will not only provide protection but will help the steroid penetrate the skin and reduce the inflammation more quickly. Another useful treatment is potassium permanganate solution. This is a purple liquid which is very effective at drying up weepy or blistering eczema. Soaking your hands and feet in the solution three or four times a day can be very soothing and will help the eczema dry up much more quickly. Potassium permanganate is available as a ready-made solution or as tablets (Permitabs®) to dissolve in water. One drawback is that it can stain skin, nails and clothing brown, so it should be demonstrated and supervised by your doctor or nurse.

In the late stages of pompholyx eczema, when the skin becomes very dry and flaky, emollients are very useful. If you are prone to developing recurrent outbreaks of pompholyx, get into the habit of using an emollient at least twice a day even when your skin is clear.

Q. Since I started an engineering job 18 months ago my hands have been gradually getting more thickened, itchy and scaly. My fingers often crack and bleed despite regular emollients. My GP has suggested a potent topical steroid but I am worried this will cause side-effects.

If you have thick, chronic eczema on your hands you will generally need a potent or very potent topical steroid such as Betnovate® or Dermovate®. Weaker topical steroids tend not to work well on thick eczema, especially on the palms, where the skin is tough. Your doctor may prescribe a potent topical steroid to use daily for between one and four weeks or sometimes longer depending on the severity of your eczema. You should put the steroid only on the affected areas of skin and not the surrounding normal skin. Remember that the skin on the backs of the hands is more delicate and will usually need shorter bursts of topical steroid compared with eczema on the palms. Cracks and fissures can be covered with simple Elastoplast, or with an adhesive tape impregnated with a moderately potent steroid called Haelan tape® (available on prescription). Continue with a regular emollient on your hands throughout the day, and use an emollient instead of soap every time you wash your hands. Very greasy emollients may make your hands slippery and may interfere with certain tasks so discuss this with your employer and doctor. Similarly, the type of gloves you wear will depend on your job although ideally cotton liners should be worn under thick, heavy work gloves if possible.

It is important that you discuss your eczema with your doctor as it sounds like your hand eczema is related to your job (occupational). Your GP is likely to refer you on to a dermatologist for patch-testing (see Chapter 11) if the problem persists.

Q. I have round patches of eczema on my lower legs which are not clearing with mild or moderate strength topical steroids. What should I use?

Some people with atopic eczema develop round patches of stubborn eczema, particularly on the legs or arms. This pattern of eczema can also occur in people without other signs of atopic eczema – it is known as discoid eczema (see Chapter 1). Discoid eczema often needs treatment with a potent topical steroid as the patches can become quite thick and inflamed. A potent topical steroid may be needed for two weeks or sometimes slightly longer, but should always be supervised by a doctor and applied only to the thick patches of eczema, not to the surrounding normal skin. You should stop your topical steroid when your symptoms have settled and the skin has returned to normal. Remember that if you have had patches of eczema for weeks or months they may leave areas of darkened skin (post-inflammatory hyperpigmentation) or lightened skin (post-inflammatory hypopigmentation) behind when they clear. These skin colour changes will fade over a few weeks and do not need treatment.

Q. Are there any alternatives to topical steroids for treating eczema?

Topical immunomodulators are a suitable alternative for selected people, as discussed in Chapter 7. Coal-tar creams and ointments can also help some people, although generally they are better for treating psoriasis (see Chapter 1) than eczema. Nevertheless, tar preparations can be useful for very thickened eczema, especially when worn under a paste bandage (see Chapter 8). Tar preparations can smell and stain your clothing, and they may irritate broken skin. Emollients should always be used along with these alternative treatments, as discussed in Chapter 5.

Basic rules for using topical steroids in eczema

1. Use the weakest topical steroid that will control your eczema.
2. Use the topical steroid intermittently for short periods when the eczema is active, followed by periods of emollient only.
3. Always use your topical steroid *as well as* – never instead of – your regular emollient.
4. Do not put your emollient and topical steroid on at the same time or you may dilute the steroid and reduce its effectiveness – allow at least half an hour between.
5. Take your tubes of topical steroid with you every time you visit the doctor or nurse so that they can see how much you have needed to use.

Chapter 7
Topical immunomodulators

Although topical steroids have been the main method of treatment for eczema for over fifty years, more recently a new type of skin treatment which contains no steroid at all has been developed. This involves using topical immunomodulators, which are so called because they modulate (or alter) the immune system in the skin. Topical immunomodulators are also sometimes known as calcineurin inhibitors because they affect the function of a protein called calcineurin in the body's cells.

There are currently two topical immunomodulators available in the UK – Protopic ointment® and Elidel cream®. They are licensed to treat atopic eczema and are generally used as second-line treatments if a person's eczema has not responded to appropriate strengths of topical steroids.

Protopic (tacrolimus)®
Protopic® (trade name) is a steroid-free ointment containing an immunomodulator called tacrolimus. Protopic® became available on prescription in the UK in April 2002. The ointment comes in two strengths, 0.1 per cent for adults and 0.03 per cent for children. It is normally used twice daily.

Elidel (pimecrolimus)®
Elidel® (trade name) is a steroid-free cream containing an immunomodulator called pimecrolimus. Elidel® became available on prescription in the UK in October 2002. It comes in one strength (1 per cent) and is normally used twice daily.

Q. How do Protopic® and Elidel® work?
The topical immunomodulators work by reducing the overactivity of the immune system. They do this by altering the action of specific cells called T-cells, which play an important role in atopic eczema. By suppressing the overactive T-cells in the skin these

treatments can reduce skin inflammation and improve the appearance and symptoms of eczema.

Q. What are the advantages of Protopic® and Elidel® over topical steroids?

The main advantage is that these treatments do not cause skin thinning. This means that Protopic® and Elidel® can be used on any part of the body, including the face, neck and skin creases. Furthermore, there is no restriction on the length of time the treatments can be used for.

Q. Can Protopic® and Elidel® be used in children as well as adults?

Yes, both Protopic® and Elidel® are licensed for use in children over the age of two years as well as adults. The lower strength of Protopic (0.03 per cent) is recommended for children.

Q. How effective are Protopic® and Elidel® in treating eczema?

In clinical trials 0.1 per cent Protopic® has proved to be as effective as a potent topical steroid. Although 0.03 per cent Protopic® is weaker it is still more effective than a mild topical steroid. Elidel® is weaker – it is less effective than a potent topical steroid but has not yet been properly compared to milder topical steroids.

Q. What are the side-effects of Protopic® and Elidel®?

One of the most common side-effects of both Protopic ointment® and Elidel cream® is a burning or tingling skin sensation after applying the treatment. This sensation usually decreases after a few days. The worse your eczema is the more likely you are to have stinging or burning. Some people's eczema becomes temporarily redder after using these treatments although worsening of the eczema is very rare. Protopic® can make your skin feel more sensitive to hot or cold temperatures, and can make you flush after drinking alcohol. Both Protopic® and Elidel® can occasionally cause acne or spots around the hair follicles (folliculitis). This is more common with Protopic® as it is available only as an ointment. Very occasionally Protopic® can cause flu-like symptoms or a headache.

Protopic® and Elidel® should not be used if your eczema is infected (see Chapter 3) as they may make the infection worse. This is because immunomodulators can alter your skin's natural resistance to infection. Protopic® and Elidel® may also slightly increase the risk of viral infections on the skin such as herpes (cold sores, chickenpox or shingles) and molluscum contagiosum (a type of wart – see Chapter 3). Therefore it is sensible to avoid topical immunomodulators if you suffer from frequent cold sores as they may encourage the virus to spread on the skin (eczema herpeticum – see Chapter 3).

Q. Could Protopic® or Elidel® affect my child's growth or development?

No, there is no evidence that either drug is absorbed in significant amounts to have any effect on growth and development or the body's natural ability to fight infections.

Q. Do Protopic® and Elidel® have any long-term side-effects?

This is still not fully known because the treatments have not been available for very long. One possible concern is whether regular use of these treatments for months or years may slightly increase the risk of skin cancer in later life. This concern has arisen because patients who take high doses of tacrolimus (the main ingredient of Protopic®) or related drugs such as ciclosporin (see Chapter 9) by mouth for many years do have an increased risk of skin cancer. This type of tablet treatment is usually used in patients who have had an organ transplant (for example, a kidney or heart transplant), where high doses of immunomodulating drugs are used to suppress the whole immune system. The body's immune system not only helps you to fight infection but also has a role in reducing the development of tumours caused by environmental damage (such as excessive sun exposure in the case of skin cancers).

Protopic® and Elidel® are very different from tablet immunomodulator drugs, and are known to have no significant effect on the general immune system. Therefore it is felt unlikely that they will be associated with any increased risk of skin cancer in the long term, and no increased risk of skin cancer has been demonstrated so far in humans. However, until Protopic® and

Elidel® have been widely used for thirty to forty years the long-term risks will not be fully known. Therefore, as a precaution, patients using Protopic® or Elidel® are advised to avoid excessive sun exposure, as sunlight is the main cause of skin cancer.

Q. Can my GP prescribe Protopic® and Elidel®?

It is recommended that these treatments are started only by doctors with a special interest and experience in managing skin diseases. Therefore your GP can start you on these treatments if he or she has a special knowledge of skin diseases. If not, he or she will refer you on to a specialist GP or dermatologist.

How to use topical immunomodulators

Q. Should I use Protopic® or Elidel® instead of my steroid creams?

Current guidelines recommend that Protopic® and Elidel® are not used as first-line treatments for people with atopic eczema. This is because in the vast majority of patients topical steroids are extremely effective and safe if used properly. Neither Protopic® or Elidel® is recommended if your eczema is mild, as low-strength topical steroids work very well in this situation.

- Protopic® is currently recommended if you have moderate to severe atopic eczema that has not been controlled with topical steroids, and where there is a risk of side-effects from further steroid use.
- Elidel® is currently recommended only for mild to moderately severe atopic eczema on the face and neck of adults and children aged between two and sixteen years who have not responded to topical steroids, and where there is a risk of side-effects from further steroid use.

Q. How should Protopic® and Elidel® be applied?

You should apply a thin layer to all affected parts of the skin twice daily. You should not apply emollients within two hours of using Protopic®, although no such restrictions are given for Elidel®. If you have had a bath or shower, make sure that your skin is completely dry before applying the treatment, as this will reduce the risk of stinging. If you are not treating your hands, wash them after you have applied Protopic® or Elidel®.

Q: Should Protopic® and Elidel® be used with suncreams?
Yes, although you should make sure that the treatments have been fully absorbed before you apply your suncreams. It is best to leave at least an hour between applying your Protopic® or Elide® and putting on your suncream.

Q. How long can I use Protopic® for?
It is recommended that you use Protopic® for up to three weeks before reducing from twice-daily to once-daily treatment until your skin clears. As with topical steroids you should stop the treatment when your skin is clear. Most people's eczema will have responded by three weeks. If your eczema is not respond-ing, Protopic® ointment may not be the best treatment for you.

Q. How long can I use Elidel® for?
Elidel is much weaker than Protopic® and there are no restric-tions on the duration of treatment. However, if your eczema has not cleared after three weeks, you should discuss with your doctor whether you need a stronger treatment.

Q. My dermatologist has prescribed me both strengths of Protopic® – should I use 0.03 per cent or 0.1 per cent first?
Adults are normally started on the stronger Protopic® prepara-tion (0.1 per cent) but should drop down to 0.03 per cent oint-ment after three weeks as their eczema improves. Only the 0.03 per cent Protopic ointment® is licensed for children (aged between two and sixteen). Children with stubborn eczema are sometimes treated with 0.1 per cent Protopic ointment® (off-licence; that is, the drug officially isn't licensed for such use but doctors may occasionally prescribe it) if 0.03 per cent Protopic® doesn't control their eczema, but this should only be on the advice of a skin specialist.

Q. Can I put my Protopic® on under my eczema bandages?
It is not recommended that either Protopic® or Elidel® is used under bandages. However, steroid creams and ointments can be

used under bandages for short periods under the supervision of your doctor or nurse.

Q. Will my child's Protopic® treatment interfere with her routine immunizations?

Although Protopic® is not known to interfere with immunizations (vaccinations), to be on the safe side it is recommended that Protopic® is stopped two weeks before immunization. For live vaccines (including measles, rubella, oral polio and BCG) Protopic® should be stopped four weeks before immunization. After both types of vaccine it is suggested that Protopic® is then not started again for three weeks. The manufacturers of Elidel® suggest that it should be stopped two weeks before vaccination, but give no specified time limit before Elidel® can be restarted.

Q. Can I use Protopic® while I am pregnant or breastfeeding?

The use of Protopic® is not recommended when you are pregnant or breastfeeding. Even though the amount absorbed into your body is very tiny, no research studies have as yet been performed in pregnant and breastfeeding mothers. Therefore, to be on the safe side it is recommended that treatment is stopped if you are pregnant or breastfeeding, although steroid creams and ointments can be used under the supervision of your doctor.

Q. Are topical immunomodulators good only for treating eczema that has already developed, or can they be used to prevent flare-ups?

This is an area where more research is needed. As with topical steroids, if you use Protopic® or Elidel® on at the first sign of your eczema coming back (red itchy skin), it may reduce the severity of your flare-up. However, it is not recommended that you carry on applying your Protopic® or Elidel® when your eczema is clear.

Using topical immunomodulators in different types of eczema

Q. I get eczema mainly around my eyelids and even if I use hydrocortisone every day it doesn't go away. What treatment should I use?

If regular mild topical steroids are not working, Protopic® and Elidel® can be useful alternatives to treat the delicate skin around the eyes. You should discuss this treatment with your doctor. Even mild steroid creams need to be used cautiously around the eyes as there is a potential risk of skin thinning, increased pressure in the eyes and even cataracts. Unfortunately, Protopic® only comes as an ointment which can look greasy on the face. However, many people find that applying the treatment only at night is enough to bring their eczema under control. Once your eczema is clear you may be able to keep it under control by using short bursts of Elidel® or Protopic® when it flares up.

Q. I have had bad eczema for many years now and my dermatologist has prescribed Protopic ointment® instead of topical steroids for my face and body. It has worked really well on my face but doesn't seem to work as well on my legs and arms. Why is this?

Protopic® can be used anywhere on the body but many people find it much less effective on thick, longstanding eczema (most common on the limbs) than on thinner patches of eczema on the face and skin creases. This is because Protopic ointment® doesn't penetrate thick eczema very easily. Many patients with lichenified eczema on the body or limbs benefit from a short course of potent topical steroid first followed by Protopic ointment® when the very thick areas have started to clear up. Discuss the problem with your dermatologist, who will advise you further.

Q. My child keeps getting weepy areas of infected eczema despite using hydrocortisone regularly. Would Protopic® or Elidel® help?

Protopic® or Elidel® aren't recommended for infected eczema as they may encourage the infection to spread. See your GP, who may prescribe a slightly stronger topical steroid to improve the eczema. If your child is getting recurrent infections your GP may also need to take a skin swab and prescribe a course of antibiotic tablets or syrup.

Q. I have had seborrhoeic eczema for three years and although antifungal creams and hydrocortisone used to work they don't keep it under control any more. Is there anything else I can try?

Yes. Protopic® and Elidel® have been used successfully in a number of people with seborrhoeic eczema, although they are currently licensed only to treat atopic eczema. Discuss these alternatives with your GP, who may refer you to your local dermatologist to talk about the treatments in more detail.

Q. Can topical immunomodulators be used to treat any other types of eczema?

Protopic® and Elidel® do seem to be effective in many types of eczema, and trials are currently under way to assess this further.

Chapter 8
Bandages

Bandages can be a very useful treatment for eczema – they protect the skin and also help other topical treatments to sink in effectively. Several different types of bandages are available. What you use depends on the type of eczema you have and what you find most comfortable. If your doctor or nurse recommends bandages it is important that you are shown how to use them safely and effectively as discussed below. We would not recommend that you use bandaging on your own without support and education from your doctor or nurse.

Wet wrap bandaging

Wet wraps are tubular cotton dressings which are applied to the skin in two layers. The bottom layer is soaked in warm water, squeezed out and then put on to the skin over an emollient or topical steroid. A dry layer of bandages is then put on top of the wet layer. Wet wraps can be worn under nightwear or ordinary clothes so they can be used during the day or night. Most patients prefer to use them for short bursts at night time, when their eczema is bad. Wet wraps are available in bandage (Tubifast®, Comfifast®, Coverflex® and ActiFast®) and garment (Comfifast®) form.

Tubular cotton bandages are prescribed in rolls of long tubular bandages which can be cut to the required length. Different lengths of bandage are cut for the arms, legs and body, and are attached together using ties (also made from the bandages). Bandages come in a range of sizes to treat patients of different ages and different parts of the body.

Tubular cotton garments are ready-made vests, tights, leggings and socks with flat seams to prevent skin irritation. Many people find them quicker and easier to use than the tubular cotton bandages.

Q. How do wet wraps work?

Wet wraps can help treat your eczema in a number of ways. They:

- keep the skin moisturized for longer
- help the creams and ointments get into the skin so that they can work more effectively
- cool and soothe the skin as the water evaporates, reducing the itch and discomfort
- cover the skin and reduce the damage from scratching
- help break the itch-scratch cycle and give the skin a chance to settle down.

Q. Can wet wraps cause any side-effects?

Side-effects are a potential problem if wet wraps are used over topical steroids, as thinning of the skin can occur more easily. However, when supervised properly the combination of topical steroids and wet wraps is an extremely useful treatment for stubborn eczema. Potent steroids should not be used under wet wraps continually for long periods of time (weeks or months) as this could lead to absorption of steroid into the bloodstream with potential effects on the rest of your body. If you are using a topical steroid under your wet wraps the steroid should only be applied to the areas of active eczema, and your emollient should be put on the non-inflamed areas of skin. Wet wraps over topical steroids should always be properly monitored by a nurse or doctor with experience in treating eczema.

It is also possible to develop an allergy to the elastic component of wet-wrap bandages or garments, although this is extremely rare. This type of allergy appears as a worsening of the eczema immediately under the bandages. If you suspect this problem, see your doctor or nurse, who can arrange patch-testing.

Using wet-wrap bandaging

Q. When should wet wraps be used?

Wet wraps are best used in patients whose eczema has not responded to standard treatment with emollients and topical steroids. They are not used as first-line treatment for eczema as they can be time-consuming and many people find them difficult to fit into their lifestyle. They also need to be supervised carefully when used over topical steroids (see above). However, many people do find them very useful, especially in short bursts to treat eczema flare-ups. Wet wraps should be started only by a doctor or nurse with experience in wet wrapping who can demonstrate the technique and teach you to use the bandages safely and effectively at home as and when required.

Q. What type of eczema are wet wraps best at treating?

Wet wraps can be used on any type of eczema as long as it is not weepy, crusty and infected. They are especially good at treating thickened (lichenified) eczema on the arms and legs as they can help the emollients and topical steroids get absorbed into the thickened skin.

Q. Are wet wraps very time-consuming?

Any form of bandaging can be time-consuming at first but as you become used to the technique it becomes much quicker. Many parents find bandaging worth the extra effort if it clears their child's skin and helps him or her sleep better. It is often best to introduce bandaging over a weekend or holiday period when there is more time and less stress.

Q. Can wet wraps be used in children and adults?

Tubifast® and Comfifast® garments are available for children from six months to fourteen years. Children, teenagers and adults can use wet-wrap bandages.

Q. How often should I use my wet wraps?

This will depend on the severity of your eczema and whether you have been told to use a topical steroid under your wet wraps – your doctor or nurse will advise you. It is usually best to start by putting the bandages on a few hours before bedtime and leaving them on for 12 to 24 hours, repeating for up to a week until the skin is clear. If you are using only emollients under your wet wraps you can continue for as long as you find helpful. However, most patients who do not require topical steroids can actually be managed without bandages.

Q. Will wet wraps help infected eczema?

No, wet wraps should not be used if your skin has open infected areas as the warmth and wetness of the bandages may make the infection worse. Once the infection has been treated wet wraps can be used.

Q. How can I keep my child still while I put her wet wraps on?

Try involving your child more. Get her to open the bandages and put them in the water, and teach her to help put her creams on. For very young children try putting the bandages on a teddy bear or doll to show them what is involved. Otherwise, put their wet wraps on in front of the television or video to distract them. Your doctor may be able to provide you with special children's leaflets designed to help your child understand wet wrapping and get more involved.

Q. My child finds the wet wraps make her chilly. Am I doing something wrong?

This is not very common, especially in young children. Try using slightly hotter water for the bandaging, and make sure the room is warm enough when you put her wet wraps on. You may also find it helpful to put the bandages on earlier in the evening so your child is not so wet when she gets into bed, and let her wear a pair of cosy pyjamas over the top.

Q. My daughter's bandages dry out very quickly and this seems to make her even more itchy. What should I do?

This is most likely to happen in hot weather over the summer months. Although you can apply the bandages twice daily it is often easier to dampen the bandages again while they are on your child, using a plant-water spray filled with warm water or a wet sponge. You can pull down the outer layer and spray the inside bandages, or simply spray both the inner and outer layers in hot weather. If she is still getting itchy it's best to stop the bandaging altogether.

Dry wrapping

A single dry layer of tubular cotton bandage or garment can also be applied over your emollient or topical steroid. This form of bandaging is sometimes helpful in teenagers and adults to help greasy moisturizers stay in place and prevent them from ruining clothing. However, in very young children dry bandages can cause overheating (especially if used at night), which can make the eczema worse.

Medicated bandages

A variety of bandages containing medicated pastes are also available for treating eczema (for example, Ichthopaste® and Calaband®). These contain substances such as calamine (soothing), zinc oxide (helps healing) and ichthammol (reduces itching). Such bandages are particularly good for softening thickened (lichenified) eczema on the arms and legs, but they should not be used on raw skin as they tend to stick to wet areas and cause further skin damage.

Q. Are paste bandages very messy and time-consuming?

Paste bandages are messier to use than wet wraps, and more time-consuming to apply. This is because they need to be pleated around the legs or arms, as you have to fold the bandage back on itself with every turn so that it doesn't cause tightness and discomfort. A layer of dry tubular, crepe, or other self-adherent bandage is then applied on top to keep the paste bandages in place and prevent staining of clothes and bedding. This whole process requires co-operation, and for this reason paste bandages are most useful in older children and adults.

Q. How long can paste bandages be left in place for?

They are usually left on for one to two days at a time before they are changed. They can be continued in this way for several weeks depending on how severe your eczema is. Your doctor or nurse will discuss this with you in more detail.

Q. My leg eczema has become very weepy and infected. Would medicated bandages help?

If your eczema is clearly infected with weeping and crusting, the infection should be treated with a course of antibiotic tablets from your doctor first. Although the bandages are mildly medicated, the warm moist environment under the bandages could encourage bacterial infection to spread. If your legs are oozing and weeping a lot, potassium permanganate (a solution available on prescription from your doctor) can be helpful if supervised by a nurse. Soak pieces of gauze in the potassium permanganate solution and wrap them around your legs for 20 minutes, three or four times a day. Remember that potassium permanganate solution can temporarily stain your skin and nails a brown colour, although this will clear over time.

Compression bandages

Compression bandages and stockings are used to treat gravitational eczema. They are elasticated and are designed to put gentle pressure on your legs to help push the blood back up your veins to your heart. As the sluggish blood flow improves so does the associated eczema. Elastic support tights or stockings are an alternative but are suitable only for mild eczema as they don't compress the legs very much; they can be bought from most pharmacies and some department stores. Compression stockings or bandages can be prescribed by your GP or dermatologist.

Before prescribing compression bandages or stockings your doctor or nurse will check the blood pressure in the arteries of your legs using a small hand-held ultrasound probe on the skin (this is called a Doppler test). This is to ensure that the blood is pumping down your legs properly. If the arteries that bring blood down your legs are blocked, compression bandages may not be suitable as they could reduce the circulation in your legs.

Q. My elderly mother was referred to our local dermatologist for her leg eczema. She has come back from hospital in compression bandages. How long will she need these for?

Compression bandages are usually used to get gravitational eczema under control. Either one or multiple layers of bandaging are applied to the legs to give stronger support than compression stockings. The bandages are usually changed once or twice a week, either at home by the district nurse or in the local community leg ulcer clinic depending on your mother's mobility. As the eczema improves your mother can be fitted with compression stockings provided she is able to use them, with nursing help arranged to supervise additional treatments if necessary.

Q. When my mother changes from compression bandages to compression stockings how long will she need to wear these for?

This very much depends on the severity of her eczema. Many people remain prone to getting gravitational eczema for the rest of their lives. This is more likely if you have bad varicose veins, or a history of deep vein thrombosis or leg ulcers. If the eczema keeps coming back every time she stops wearing her compression stockings, she should ideally get into the habit of wearing them every day, both to keep the eczema controlled and to reduce the risk of a leg ulcer developing.

Q. When should compression stockings be worn?

Compression stockings should be put on first thing in the morning before getting out of bed (before any fluid has had a chance to build up), and taken off before going to bed. Ordinary stockings or tights can be worn over the top if wished.

Chapter 9
Light therapy and tablet treatment

If your eczema doesn't settle with creams, ointments and bandages, other treatments can help. For some people a course of light treatment can be very beneficial to bring the condition back under control. For others a course of tablet treatment to suppress the immune system is more effective. However, all the treatments discussed in this chapter carry more potential for side-effects compared with topical treatments and bandages. For this reason your doctor will recommend these treatments only if your eczema has not responded to other therapies.

Light therapy (or phototherapy)

Many people find that their eczema improves when they go on a sunny holiday and this is related to the beneficial effects of sunlight on skin inflammation. Ultraviolet light (which is found in sunlight) is used by dermatologists to treat many inflammatory skin diseases, including eczema and psoriasis. Ultraviolet light can be divided into two different wavelengths called ultraviolet A (UVA) and ultraviolet B (UVB). Artificial forms of both UVA and UVB can be used to treat people with eczema.

Q. What does light therapy involve?

Light therapy is usually carried out in a hospital dermatology department. The ultraviolet light is produced in a big cabinet which you stand in; this looks like an upright sun bed but is actually very different from a standard sun bed. Treatment is usually carried out two or three times a week for six to twelve weeks (sometimes longer). While you are standing in the cabinet you will need to wear goggles to protect your eyes from the light. Each individual treatment takes only a few minutes.

Q. What is the difference between UVA and UVB light therapy?

UVA alone is not very effective at treating eczema so it is given with a medicine called psoralen. This treatment is called PUVA (**P**soralen and **UVA**). Psoralens are naturally occurring chemicals which make your skin more sensitive to light. The psoralen can either be taken in tablet form two hours before your UVA treatment, or you can soak in a bath containing psoralen before your light treatment. If you have tablet PUVA you will need to wear dark sunglasses for the rest of the day (24 hours) until the psoralen has cleared from your body, as your skin will temporarily be more sensitive to natural sunlight.

UVB light is usually given three times a week. No tablets or baths are required before treatment, and goggles need to be worn only inside the light cabinet and not afterwards.

Q. Is light treatment uncomfortable?

No, the treatment should not be uncomfortable or painful, although you may feel a little hot or itchy during or after therapy. Some people feel a little nauseous after their psoralen tablets, although this can be reduced by taking the tablets with food. Occasionally, light therapy can make your eczema flare up slightly at the beginning of the treatment course but this usually settles with continued treatment.

Q. What are the possible side-effects of ultraviolet light therapy?

Short-term side effects: As with sun exposure, ultraviolet light therapy carries a small risk of skin burning (like sunburn). This is not common because at the beginning of treatment only small doses of light are given, with gradual increases depending on your skin's response. Light therapy can also cause itching, although this usually settles quickly after treatment.

Long-term side effects: Although ultraviolet light is good at settling down inflamed skin, too much light can be bad for you. As with sunlight, too much ultraviolet light treatment can increase the long-term risk of skin cancer and premature ageing of the skin. The risk depends on the amount of light treatment you have, but it is highest in people who have had numerous courses of ultraviolet light treatment (more than 150–200 treatment sessions).

Q. Can light treatment be used in children as well as adults?

Yes, as long as the child is old enough to stand in the light cabinet by him- or herself without getting frightened. However, because of the small increased risk of skin cancer and because children's delicate skin is more susceptible to sun damage than adults' skin it is used in children only if other treatments have failed.

Q. How long will the effects of light treatment last after I've finished the course?

This is very variable. Many people find the improvement in their skin lasts for weeks or months after a course of treatment. Light treatment can be useful to break the chronic cycle of itching and scratching which often leads to thick stubborn eczema. Once this has cleared many people find it much easier to stay on top of their condition by promptly treating any new patches of eczema with topical treatment before the eczema gets out of control again.

Tablet treatment

Steroid tablets

Steroids can be taken by mouth as well as in cream or ointment form. When given in tablet form, steroids suppress your body's whole immune system, reducing any inflammation in your body, including your skin. Steroid tablets are sometimes used to treat asthma as they can also reduce any inflammation in your lungs and airways. Patients with eczema and asthma often find their eczema temporarily improves while they are on steroids for their asthma.

The most commonly prescribed oral steroid is prednisolone. When given by mouth steroids are very effective for treating eczema, but unfortunately have many side-effects that make them very unsuitable for long-term treatment. Steroid tablets are generally used only in short bursts of one to two weeks to bring severe eczema back under control and should never be used over prolonged periods for eczema except in exceptional circumstances (under the supervision of a dermatologist). A typical course of oral steroids in an adult would be 20–40 mg per day for one to two weeks.

Q. What are the possible side-effects of steroid tablets?

Side-effects are most likely to be a problem if you are taking steroid tablets for several weeks or months. A course of oral steroids for one to two weeks is much less likely to cause problems, although users should be aware of the risk of indigestion (or even stomach ulceration) and increased susceptibility to infections. Other potential side-effects include thinning of the bones, weight gain, growth reduction (in children), increased blood pressure and mood changes. Oral steroids can increase blood sugar levels so they need to be used very carefully if you are diabetic. Very high doses of oral steroids can give you stretch marks, swelling of the face and upper body, and acne.

Q. Are there any special precautions I should take while I am on oral steroids?

Your doctor should give you a steroid treatment card which you should carry with you while you are on treatment. This will list the important precautions you need to take while you are on steroid tablets, and also alert other people to the fact that you are on oral steroids if you become ill while you are on treatment. The steroid treatment card carries a warning that:

- you should contact your doctor immediately if you become ill, or come into contact with anyone who has an infectious disease
- if you have never had chickenpox (and are therefore not immune to the virus) you should avoid close contact with people who have chickenpox or shingles. If you do come into contact with chickenpox or shingles while on oral steroids or within three months of finishing the course see your doctor immediately (you may need a protective injection within three days of exposure)
- you should not stop taking your steroid tablets suddenly if you have been on them for more than three weeks. Your doctor will advise you on how to reduce the dose gradually. This is because synthetic steroid tablets temporarily reduce your body's natural

production of steroids (which are important to help your body work properly). Gradual reduction of your steroid tablets will allow your body to safely start making its own steroids again.

Q. Can steroid tablets be used to treat children with eczema?

Steroid tablets are generally best avoided in children and adolescents if possible as they can affect the child's growth. If a short course of steroids is needed, it is unlikely to be associated with any serious long-term side-effects. Your doctor will always weigh up the risks and benefits to your individual child.

Q. My GP has put me on a two-week course of prednisolone for my eczema. Can I use a steroid ointment at the same time?

Yes, it is a good idea to continue with a steroid ointment (as prescribed by your doctor) as you can target the worst parts of your skin and help the steroid tablets get your eczema back under control. Remember that you need to get into the habit of using your steroid ointment regularly on an intermittent basis (under your doctor's guidance) as topical steroids are a much more suitable maintenance treatment than prednisolone.

Ciclosporin

Ciclosporin is a very effective drug for people with severe eczema that has not responded to creams, ointments or bandages. Ciclosporin is an immunosuppressant drug; it suppresses the body's immune system in a slightly different way to oral steroids. Ciclosporin is widely used in patients who have had an organ transplant (for example, kidney, heart, liver or bone marrow transplant) to prevent organ rejection. In the treatment of skin diseases such as eczema much lower doses of ciclosporin are needed, and it is generally considered a more suitable long-term treatment than steroid tablets. Nevertheless, ciclosporin is a very powerful drug with many side-effects and should be used to treat eczema only under the close supervision of a skin specialist.

Q. How effective is ciclosporin in treating eczema?

At least nine out of ten patients treated with ciclosporin will notice a significant improvement in their eczema. The itching, soreness and redness usually clear significantly over two to six weeks, and most patients find their overall quality of life improves greatly while they are on the treatment.

Q. How does ciclosporin work?

Ciclosporin alters the action of T-cells (important cells in the immune system) in the skin and blood. It stops the T-cells producing the chemical messengers that cause skin inflammation. The mechanism of action of ciclosporin is similar to that of the topical immunomodulators Protopic® and Elidel® (see Chapter 7), although it is usually more effective.

Q. What are the possible side-effects of ciclosporin?

Ciclosporin has many potential side-effects but these can usually be managed or avoided with regular monitoring.

Kidney damage: The most important potential side-effect is a reduction in the efficiency of your kidneys. The chances of this occurring increase the longer you take the drug and the higher the dose you take. Your doctor will need to take blood tests to monitor your kidneys, initially every two weeks and then approximately every two months while you are on ciclosporin. If your kidney tests change the dose can be reduced and the test results usually return to normal. However, if the tests remain abnormal ciclosporin will need to be stopped in order to prevent permanent kidney damage.

High blood pressure: Ciclosporin can raise your blood pressure. Your doctor will check your blood pressure regularly while you are on treatment and reduce the dose or start you on a blood pressure tablet if necessary.

Other, less common, side-effects include tiredness, nausea (feeling sick), gum swelling, shakiness, pins and needles or burning sensations in the hands and feet, increased hair growth and raised cholesterol. Patients who are on ciclosporin for years (especially transplant patients) have a slightly increased risk of skin cancers, although in atopic eczema ciclosporin is usually used only for a few months at a time. If you have had a serious cancer in the past (internal cancer or skin cancer) ciclosporin may not be suitable for you as alterations in the immune system may affect cancer growth. As with most drugs ciclosporin should also be avoided in pregnancy.

Q. Can ciclosporin be used in children?

Although ciclosporin is not licensed for the treatment of eczema in children under the age of 16 years, it is widely used by dermatologists (off-licence) to treat children with very severe eczema if other standard treatments have failed and their quality of life is being severely affected by the disease. It should not be used to treat children with eczema outside the setting of a hospital dermatology department.

Q. Should I carry on using my topical steroids at the same time as my ciclosporin?

Your doctor will usually ask you to continue with supervised amounts of topical steroids, although lower strengths are often needed if you are taking ciclosporin. By continuing with your topical treatment you can reduce the amount of ciclosporin that you need. You should also continue to use your regular emollient. Occasionally your doctor will prescribe ciclosporin to give your skin a rest from topical steroids, especially if you have been using excessive amounts of potent steroids for long periods of time. If this is the case you should just use your emollient. Discuss your treatment with your doctor if you are at all unsure.

Q. How long can ciclosporin be used for?

Ideally, ciclosporin should be used for short periods of up to two months at a time to bring your eczema under control. Sometimes the eczema can flare up quickly after stopping ciclosporin, but in many people the disease can stay well controlled for months or longer after the vicious cycle of itching and scratching has been broken. A small number of adult patients with very severe eczema need to take ciclosporin for several months or even years, although the longer it is taken the more potential there is for side-effects.

Q. Could ciclosporin interact with any of my other medicines?

Yes. If you are on ciclosporin always check with your doctor before taking any other tablets as they may interact. Your doctor should give you a list of all drugs that may interact. These include antibiotics such as erythromycin, painkillers and some blood pressure tablets, all of which can increase the levels of ciclosporin in your blood and increase the risk of side-effects. Grapefruit juice should also be avoided as it can raise the blood levels of ciclosporin.

Azathioprine

Azathioprine is an immunosuppressant drug that can be used as an alternative to ciclosporin for the treatment of severe eczema. Azathioprine has been used effectively for many years to treat patients who have received organ transplants. The drug is also used to treat a number of other skin conditions as well as eczema, but its use needs to be closely supervised by a skin specialist.

Q. How effective is azathioprine in treating eczema?

Azathioprine has not been as widely studied as ciclosporin for the treatment of atopic eczema. It is very effective in reducing skin inflammation and helping get eczema under control, but some people find the side-effects (see below) troublesome. It is a useful drug for people with severe eczema who cannot take ciclosporin for other medical reasons such as high blood pressure.

Q. How does azathioprine work?

Azathioprine interferes with cell division and replication. It reduces the activity of T-cells (cells of the immune system), which are involved in causing eczema.

Q. What are the possible side-effects of azathioprine?

The main side-effect of azathioprine is on the bone marrow (where blood cells are made), which can cause anaemia and increased risk of infection, bleeding and bruising. Azathioprine can also occasionally cause inflammation in the liver or pancreas. You will need blood tests to monitor for these side-effects every week for the first month, and then every three months or more while you remain on the treatment.

Other side-effects include nausea (feeling sick), vomiting and diarrhoea. Patients who are on azathioprine for years (especially transplant patients) have an increased risk of skin cancers, as with ciclosporin. If you had a serious cancer (internal cancer or skin cancer) in the past, azathioprine may not be a suitable treatment for you as alterations in the immune system may affect cancer growth. As with most drugs azathioprine should also be avoided in pregnancy.

Q. Can azathioprine be used in children?

As with ciclosporin, azathioprine is not licensed for the treatment of eczema in children under the age of 16 years. It is more commonly used to treat adults, but it is occasionally used by dermatologists (off-licence) to treat children with very severe eczema if other standard treatments have failed and their quality of life is being severely affected by the disease. As with ciclosporin it should not be used to treat children with eczema outside the setting of a hospital dermatology department.

Q. How long can azathioprine be used for?

Ideally, azathioprine should be taken for a few months to get your eczema under control rather than as a long-term treatment. In adults occasionally the drug is needed for months or even years although the benefits always need to be carefully weighed up against the long-term risk of side-effects such as skin cancer.

Q. Can azathioprine interact with other medications?

Yes. If you are on azathioprine always check with your doctor before taking any other tablets as they may interact. Your doctor should give you a list of all drugs that may interact. These include allopurinol (for gout), warfarin (for thinning the blood) and some antibiotics, painkillers and blood pressure tablets.

Other tablet treatments for eczema

Antihistamines

Antihistamines are often prescribed in patients with eczema but there is not much evidence that they actually reduce itching. Their main use in people with eczema is as a sedative, to help them get some sleep at night. They are best taken an hour before bedtime. A short course of antihistamines can be useful during an eczema flare-up when night-time scratching and sleep disturbance can be a real problem. However, antihistamines should not be used as a substitute for other eczema treatments as by themselves they will not improve underlying eczema.

Q. Are some antihistamines more effective than others?

Many different antihistamines are available either from your pharmacist or on prescription from your GP. Many of the newer antihistamines, such as Neoclarityn® (desloratadine) and Zirtek® (cetirizine), are specially designed not to make you sleepy (nonsedating). Although these newer preparations are useful in other conditions such as hayfever and urticaria, they aren't very effective at helping people get to sleep. The older antihistamines, such as Piriton®, Vallergan®, Atarax® and Phenergan®, are more helpful in people with eczema as they are quite sedating. Remember that sedating antihistamines may affect your ability to perform skilled tasks such as driving, and their sedative effects will be enhanced by alcohol so heavy drinking should be avoided. Some people find they still feel sleepy when they wake up. If this is a problem try taking the tablet earlier in the evening.

Q. Can antihistamines be used in children?

Yes, certain antihistamines are licensed for use in children, but they should only be used for short periods during flare-ups while waiting for creams and ointments to take effect. Remember that they may make your child feel sleepy in the morning and this could affect his or her school work. If this is a problem give the antihistamine tablets or syrup earlier in the evening, or reduce the dose.

Antibiotic tablets

Antibiotic tablets are needed only if eczema becomes infected with bacteria. The most common antibiotic tablets to be prescribed in people with eczema are flucloxacillin and erythromycin. If your eczema becomes very inflamed and weepy, or the skin develops yellow crusts or pus-filled spots, it is likely that you have a bacterial infection. See your doctor or nurse if this occurs, and refer to Chapter 3 for more information about infected eczema.

Antiviral tablets

Antiviral tablets are used to treat eczema herpeticum, a secondary infection caused by the *herpes* virus, which can spread over the skin very rapidly in people with eczema. The most common antiviral tablet is aciclovir, given five times daily for five days. It is likely that you have eczema herpeticum if you develop many small, round, painful ulcers on top of your eczema, especially if you or someone you have been in contact with has recently had cold sores. See your doctor if you suspect eczema herpeticum, and refer to Chapter 3 for more information about the condition.

Antifungal tablets

Very occasionally a short course of antifungal tablets (such as itraconazole) is used to treat adults with severe seborrhoeic eczema that has not responded to simple creams and shampoos (see Chapter 6). However, antifungal tablets are not used to treat other types of eczema. Antifungal tablets are not suitable for long-term use as they can occasionally be associated with side-effects such as liver inflammation. Usually these tablets are started by a dermatologist, who would also exclude any associated conditions that may be stopping the seborrhoeic eczema from responding to standard treatment.

Chapter 10
Alternative treatments and interventions

This chapter looks at treatment approaches for eczema that don't usually form part of conventional medical therapy. This includes a wide range of complementary therapies, as well as other non-pharmacological approaches (that is, those not based on drug treatment). In general there is much less research evidence to show that these treatments are effective, although they certainly do seem to benefit some people with eczema.

Complementary therapies
A number of practitioners in the UK and abroad offer complementary treatments for a variety of medical conditions including eczema. Complementary medical practitioners are often not medically trained and usually work privately outside the NHS, although links between conventional and complementary medicine are expanding. Some complementary therapies are now available through selected GPs and hospital skin departments – ask your doctor for more details. Increasing numbers of people with eczema are trying complementary therapies for various reasons, including concern about side-effects from conventional treatments, and increased access to such therapies through the Internet and the media. People should be aware that some complementary practitioners are much better than others and unfortunately regulation of complementary practice is not yet satisfactory. In safe hands many people do benefit from these therapies, although unfortunately many others find very little improvement in their skin. A small number of people actually become much worse after using complementary therapy, especially when they are advised to stop all conventional treatments during therapy. For this reason it is very important to liaise closely with your GP or dermatologist if you are considering any

of these therapies. Most NHS doctors and nurses will be very supportive in helping you to explore all possible avenues of treatment for your eczema, providing you are fully aware of the risks and benefits involved.

Q. Are complementary therapies the same as alternative therapies?

Strictly speaking, the term 'complementary' means that the therapy is used *alongside* conventional treatment, whereas 'alternative' therapies are used *instead of* conventional treatments. Practitioners may sometimes recommend the same treatment as an alternative therapy in one person and a complementary therapy in another. The therapies discussed below should be used to complement your conventional treatments. Patients have become severely ill on stopping their conventional treatments (and sometimes even need to be admitted to hospital) because their alternative therapies alone have failed to control their eczema.

Q. Why are complementary therapies not more widely available on the NHS?

Conventional medical treatments are based on scientific research studies and well-documented experience from clinical practice. This provides doctors and nurses with accurate information about the benefits and safety of different treatments, and therapies that don't benefit the majority of patients are usually not licensed or given NHS funding. Unfortunately, in the past many complementary practitioners have not been prepared to organize good-quality research studies to prove the benefit of their treatments, or quantify the potential risks. This is slowly changing. As more complementary therapies are put through the same vigorous assessments as conventional medicines, they are likely to become more widely accepted in the NHS, providing they can be shown to be safe and effective.

Q. How can I find a good complementary practitioner?

The Skin Care Campaign and the Royal College of Nursing have put together a very helpful checklist to consider when choosing a complementary practitioner.

1.a. Questions to ask of complementary or non-orthodox practitioners:

- What are his or her qualifications and how long was the training?
- Is he or she a member of a recognized registered body with a code of practice?
- Can you obtain the address and telephone number of this body so that you can check?
- Is the therapy available on the NHS?
- Can your GP delegate care to this practitioner?
- Does he or she keep your GP informed in the same way that a hospital consultant would?
- Is this the most suitable complementary medicine for your condition?
- Are the records confidential?
- What is the cost of the treatment?
- How many treatments will be needed?
- Does the practitioner have insurance cover?

b. Then ask yourself whether the practitioner:

- answered your questions clearly and to your satisfaction
- gave you information to look through at your leisure
- conducted him- or herself in a professional manner
- made excessive claims about the treatment? (Remember, eczema is usually controllable rather than curable.)

2. It is best to avoid any practitioner who:

- claims to be able to completely 'cure' your eczema
- advises you to stop your conventional treatment without consulting your GP
- makes you feel uncomfortable – a good relationship is essential to ensure full benefit from treatment.

3. Finally, do you feel you can trust the answers to the above questions and how would you set about making sure?

If you are unsure, think carefully before you proceed – the treatment on offer may be too good to be true.

Q. How can I find out more about complementary medicine for my eczema?

The National Eczema Society (see Resources at the end of this book) produces a very helpful list of organizations that can put you in touch with registered practitioners in or near your area.

Chinese herbal medicine

Chinese herbal medicine consists of plant extracts of various kinds that can be taken by mouth or put on the skin in cream or ointment form. Oral preparations are usually prepared by boiling the herbs in water and drinking the liquid (which often tastes unpleasant) like a tea. Various parts of plants can be used, including the roots, bark, stem, seeds, flowers and leaves. Practitioners usually use different combinations of herbs for different individuals, depending on their assessment of a patient's skin condition. Chinese herbs appear to work by altering the immune system and decreasing inflammation.

Q. How effective are Chinese herbs in treating people with eczema?

As with many complementary therapies there haven't been enough good-quality research studies to show whether Chinese herbs are effective in the majority of people. Those studies that have been performed in patients with atopic eczema have shown conflicting results. A proportion of people do seem to benefit from the treatment although many others don't. Some people actually become ill as a result of treatment. Many of these research studies used a Chinese herbal product called Zemaphyte® which was available in the past on the NHS but which is no longer being manufactured.

Q. Are Chinese herbs more effective if taken by mouth rather than as a cream?

There is not enough evidence to answer this question. Both oral and topical preparations containing many different combinations of herbs have been used in many different kinds of patients, which has made it difficult to compare different preparations accurately. How your eczema responds to the treatments is very individual. However, herbal tablets have more potential side-effects than creams as they are absorbed into your circulation and can affect other parts of your body as well as your skin.

Q. I thought all herbal treatments were safe – after all, they are just based on plants aren't they?

Just because something is labelled 'herbal' does not mean that it is safe. Although herbs are plants, you must remember that many plants are poisonous to humans. Many conventional medicines have been developed from plants, including morphine for pain (from poppies) and digoxin for heart disease (from foxgloves) – drugs that can be extremely dangerous or even fatal if taken in the wrong dose.

Q. What are the potential side-effects of Chinese herbal medicines?

Common side-effects of Chinese herbal tablets include stomach upsets, bloatedness, headaches and dizziness. More serious side-effects that have been reported include liver failure, kidney failure, allergic reactions and even death. Side-effects are less common with Chinese herbal creams, although skin irritation and allergy can occur.

As with most other tablets, herbal tablets should be avoided in pregnancy, and should not be taken if you have any serious liver or kidney disease.

If you think that you may have suffered a reaction to a herbal remedy you should stop it and tell your doctor or pharmacist, as there are systems in place for reporting any concerns.

Q. I have heard that many Chinese herbal medicines are contaminated with dangerous ingredients. Is this true?

Yes, worryingly there have been an increasing number of reports of Chinese herbal medicines containing dangerous or prohibited ingredients. This problem has been identified in Chinese herbs that patients have bought from a variety of sources including practitioners, herbal clinics, market stalls and mail-order and overseas companies. These ingredients include:

- prohibited herbs, such as Aristolochia, which can cause kidney failure and cancer

- toxic products, such as mercury, lead and arsenic
- biological products, such as human placenta and excreta from bats
- prescription medicines, such as strong steroids.

It may be very difficult for you to tell exactly what is in your herbal tablets. If you plan to try Chinese herbs, follow the guidelines above when choosing a practitioner, and report any concerns to your family doctor.

Q. My friend has suggested I try a Chinese herbal cream for my eczema. Surely this is safe?

Not necessarily. In a recent study in Birmingham the majority of herbal creams that patients were using were actually found to contain topical steroids. Some of the creams tested, including Wau Wa cream and Muijiza cream, actually contained clobetasol propionate (Dermovate®), which is a very potent topical steroid that can cause side-effects such as skin thinning if not used carefully. This is ironic as some patients turn to 'herbal creams' because of their concern about topical steroids. Many herbal creams are perfectly safe, but unfortunately because there are so many contaminated preparations around it is difficult to reassure you – if you are worried don't use the cream and discuss the problem with your doctor.

Q. I have been giving my son Chinese herbal tea, which seems to have helped his eczema slightly. Should he be having any tests to monitor the treatment?

Yes. He should be having blood tests to check his liver and kidneys as the herbs can sometimes cause inflammation of the liver (hepatitis) and occasionally damage the kidneys. Remember also that the long-term side-effects of oral Chinese herbal medicines have not been well studied, so close monitoring is essential.

Other herbal medicines

A number of other herbal treatments have been used to treat eczema but there is very little evidence that they are of benefit. They include arnica, chamomile and tea tree oil. These herbs are usually used as creams and are generally well tolerated but can sometimes cause skin irritation or an allergic contact dermatitis.

Q. What regulations are in place to ensure that no dangerous herbal medicines are sold to the public?

Some herbal medicines are licensed in much the same way as other drugs available on the NHS. Other herbal medicines do not currently need to be licensed. For these unlicensed herbal remedies no specific safeguards on quality and safety are in place. There is also currently not enough information for the public about the safe use of unlicensed herbal products. This arrangement gives you choice, but not enough protection.

The Medicines and Healthcare products Regulatory Agency (MHRA) is a Department of Health agency which oversees the safety of medicines in the UK. It is currently monitoring the safety of herbal treatments and looking at ways of improving their regulation to ensure that side-effects are avoided. Useful information about herbal treatment safety can be found on the MHRA website (see Resources).

Homeopathy

Homeopathy is a therapy based on the principle of similars – 'like cures like'. The basis of this treatment is a belief that a substance that can cause certain symptoms in a healthy person can cure similar symptoms in an unhealthy person. Homeopathy claims to aid and stimulate the body's own defence and immune processes to treat or prevent a range of medical conditions, including eczema. Homeopathic medicines are derived from a variety of plants and minerals, and are normally taken in the form of tablets. These medicines are prescribed to fit each individual's needs, and are given in much smaller doses than traditional medicines. In fact, the treatments are often diluted so much that virtually no active treatment is left in the preparation – normally one part of the remedy to around 1,000,000,000,000 parts of water. This has led to much scepticism among conventional doctors, as there is little scientific basis to how such diluted treatments could work.

Q. Is there any evidence to support the use of homeopathy in eczema?

The evidence supporting the use of homeopathy in eczema is very limited but the Centre of Evidence-Based Dermatology (based in Nottingham) is currently collaborating with the Faculty of Homeopathy and the British Homeopathic Association to conduct further research into the use of homeopathy for the treatment of childhood eczema.

Q. Can homeopathy be dangerous?

No, this is very unlikely. However, if you have severe eczema and stop all your conventional treatments while having your homeopathy there is a significant risk that your eczema will flare up badly.

Aromatherapy

Aromatherapy involves the use of essential oils which are extracted from the roots, flowers and leaves of perfumed plants. The oils can be massaged into the skin, added to your bath water or inhaled. Although aromatherapy is usually very safe, occasionally the essential oils can cause skin irritation or allergy. There is very little evidence that aromatherapy is an effective treatment for eczema. When oils that are massaged into the skin are used, the massage itself may be more beneficial than the oils. Most people find aromatherapy very relaxing, and by reducing your stress levels you may feel much better even if your eczema doesn't necessarily improve significantly.

Massage

Massage may be helpful in people with eczema by leading to a reduction in stress levels and enabling patients to relax. There are limited studies in relation to massage and eczema, although one study showed that massage made parents and their children less anxious and more able to cope with the condition. Parents can very easily be taught to massage their children, and this can have a beneficial effect on their children's eczema in some cases. However, the technique needs to be gentle when used in people with eczema, and areas of broken skin should be avoided. The skin should ideally be massaged in a downwards direction as you would do when putting on your emollients (see Chapter 5), to avoid the hair follicles becoming inflamed. Perfumed oils that may irritate the skin are generally best avoided, although massaging with your emollients can be beneficial.

Reflexology

Reflexology is a complementary therapy that involves working on a person's feet. It is based on the belief that certain areas of the foot correspond to particular parts of the body, and that tension in a part of the foot reflects an ailment in the corresponding part of the body. Reflexologists uses their hands to detect subtle changes in specific points on the feet, to which they then apply pressure. A treatment session usually lasts for about one hour, and practitioners will often recommend a course of treatment. Reflexology can be a useful technique for counteracting stress, which may in turn help some people's eczema, although again the technique has not been proven to be effective in treating eczema.

Hypnotherapy

Hypnotherapy is a technique which uses relaxation and mental imagery. It aims to let your subconscious mind respond to a therapist's suggestions without your normal 'thinking' conscious state of mind getting in the way. In this relaxed state the therapist can suggest ideas, concepts and lifestyle adaptations which are likely to stick in your mind and potentially give long-term health benefits. It has been used to try to reduce habit scratching in children, and in some people it does seem to reduce skin discomfort and ease the desire to itch. Modified forms of hypnotherapy involving story-telling can be used in young children, and they often find the therapy very enjoyable as it uses their imagination. For children and adults with eczema some benefits have been demonstrated in a few small studies, although again the overall research evidence is very limited.

Acupuncture

Acupuncture is a therapy based on ancient Chinese medicine which involves the insertion of fine, sterile needles into various points of the body. Central to the technique is the belief that your health is dependent on the body's motivating energy (known as *Qi*) moving in a smooth and balanced way through a series of channels beneath the skin. It is thought that imbalances in the flow of this energy can lead to illnesses such as eczema. By inserting fine needles into the channels of energy, the aim of the acupuncturist is to stimulate the body's own healing response and help restore its natural balance. It is not usually painful but the needles may give a pinprick or tingling sensation when inserted. There is very little scientific evidence that acupuncture can help eczema, although it is usually very safe if carried out by a trained practitioner.

General advice with complementary therapies

1. Don't try many different complementary therapies at once: if you get better you won't know which one has helped.
2. Make sure that you visit a registered practitioner.
3. Tell your doctor or eczema team if you are undergoing any form of complementary treatment in case it interacts with any of your conventional treatments. This is particularly important if you are on any tablets such as steroids or ciclosporin as some herbal treatments can alter the level of these drugs in your blood.

Psychological approaches

A number of psychological therapies have been used to treat patients with eczema. Certainly psychological and emotional factors do seem to play a role in the disease. Behavioural modification techniques have been used successfully in a number of patients to help break the cycle of itching and scratching which can prevent the skin from healing. These techniques are usually performed by a clinical psychologist and are available on the NHS in many areas – ask your doctor or eczema team for more details. One of the most widely used behavioural techniques for eczema is habit reversal.

Habit reversal

Habit reversal is a modified behavioural technique which teaches patients to recognize the habit of picking or scratching the skin. Although scratching in atopic eczema begins as a conscious reaction to itch, later the behaviour becomes unconscious and is stimulated by a wide variety of situations and activities, without itch necessarily being involved. Habit reversal works by making you aware of your behaviour so it is conscious again. It can help you identify the situations that provoke scratching and adopt strategies to deal with these situations. Habit reversal has been used successfully in a number of other areas such as weight loss, smoking cessation and nail-biting, and has shown promising results so far in people with eczema.

Q. I know I am always scratching my eczema subconsciously and am interested in finding out more about habit reversal. What does it involve?

This type of therapy does not suit everyone. You must want to give up the scratching and have time to commit to the programme – it usually involves about six appointments. Scratching (including all touching, rubbing and picking of the skin) is recorded daily for several days, using a tally counter. During this time you will be asked to identify activities or emotions that make you scratch more. Alternative 'safe behaviours' are suggested every time you get the urge to scratch. The technique does require the support of family and friends to help with the tally counting (for example, saying 'click' if they see you scratching). It can be used with children but their age and development is an important consideration; in young children it requires close monitoring in conjunction with techniques such as distraction and rewards for applying their creams.

Habit reversal is always combined with conventional treatment of eczema; there is no point in trying to stop you itching if you have uncontrolled inflamed eczema. Throughout the sessions both the psychological and conventional aspects of your treatment are discussed regularly and reviewed, helping you recognize how your eczema looks and feels and when to intervene with treatments.

Dietary interventions

The role of food allergies and specific dietary manipulation in the treatment of eczema is discussed in detail in Chapters 10 and 11.

Exclusion diets

Removal of foods from your diet should never be done without discussion with your doctor as it can result in serious deficiencies of vitamins and nutrients. Your doctor can put you in touch with a dietician to supervise dietary manipulation if you would like to pursue this line of treatment.

Vitamin and mineral supplements

There is no medical evidence that supplements with vitamins and minerals such as vitamin E, pyridoxine, selenium or zinc have any overall benefit in people with eczema, and such supplements should not be required providing you are on a healthy, balanced diet.

Evening primrose oil

Evening primrose oil contains essential fatty acids and has been widely used in the past to treat atopic eczema. Treatment was based on the theory that deficiency of fatty acids may contribute to skin inflammation and skin barrier damage in people with eczema. The emergence of this natural plant oil extract in the early 1980s was well received as a possible alternative to conventional treatment. Interest was fuelled because evening primrose oil extract was shown to cause few side-effects and there was a plausible mechanism to explain why supplementation with this essential fatty acid might work in atopic eczema. However, over recent years numerous large studies have rigorously evaluated its effectiveness for atopic eczema and concluded that overall there is no evidence that it is beneficial. As a result the UK Medicines Control Agency has withdrawn the product licence for its use in atopic eczema, and it is no longer available on the NHS. No safety issues have been associated with its withdrawal, and evening primrose oil is still available in health food shops for those who wish to take a dietary supplement.

Probiotics

Probiotics are 'friendly' bacteria that are thought to help your intestines to work properly. Supplements and foods containing probiotics are available from health food shops, supermarkets and pharmacies. They are thought to be beneficial because healthy people's guts contain many harmless bacteria. It has been suggested that people with atopic diseases such as atopic eczema have an imbalance of bacteria in their guts, with not enough friendly bacteria (such as *Lactobacillus* and *Bifidobacterium*). It is thought that this makes their guts more 'leaky', allowing substances to get absorbed from the gut into the circulation more easily and trigger allergy or inflammation. Attempts have been made to prevent the development of atopic eczema in children with a family history of atopy by administering probiotics to mothers during pregnancy or breastfeeding, or to the new-born infants. Some evidence has been found that probiotics may reduce the development of eczema when used in this way although further studies are needed to confirm their benefit. There is as yet no convincing evidence that probiotics help children or adults with established atopic eczema. Although probiotics are generally well tolerated and safe, the preparations available do vary in quality, and they can occasionally cause stomach upsets.

Salt baths

Salt water has been used for years to treat a number of skin diseases including eczema. Although little scientific evidence is available that salt water improves eczema, there are many reports of patients finding it helpful, and many doctors do recommend salt water baths alongside conventional treatments. Salt water can have a weak antiseptic action and it can be particularly helpful if the eczema is oozing a lot or if secondary infection is a problem. The salt water may help to draw out excess fluid that has accumulated in little water blisters in the skin. Salt water may also help to heal any minor cuts and scratches.

Q. My child's eczema always seems to clear up when he swims in the sea on holiday. Is this because of the salt water?

Many parents find their child's eczema improves on seaside holidays. The sea could certainly be playing a role, but other factors such as the effects of sunshine, reduced stress levels and reduced exposure to house dust mite could be equally important. Many patients have reported benefits from holidays in the Dead Sea, where the combined effect of sunlight and salt water seems to be particularly effective.

Q. I would like to try salt baths for my son. How do I go about it?

You should try to mimic the concentration of sea water as closely as possible. Sea salt can be quite expensive and it is important that you shop around to get the best bulk buy as you will need quite a lot of salt to get a decent concentration in the bath.

You will need to use around a 20 fl oz jug of sea salt per 3 gallon bucket of water in order to achieve a similar concentration to sea water. It is important to use sea salt rather than other types of chemical salts, and to ensure that the salt is fully dissolved in warm water before pouring it into the bath. It is usually easier to pour the salt into the bottom of the bucket and dissolve it in a little warm water before pouring it into the bath. Around three buckets will usually be enough for your child to soak in.

If your child has a lot of broken skin the salt water (or indeed any type of water) can cause temporary stinging. It is important that the broken skin is first treated with steroid creams and moisturizers before introducing the bathing. If your child hates the bathing process, there is little point in persisting with it as you will simply create resentment and further difficulties when it comes to applying other treatments.

Q. How often should salt baths be used?

There is no right or wrong answer although twice weekly is a good idea to start with. If you find you benefit from it, the frequency can be increased. It should be emphasized that salt-water bathing should form part of your conventional eczema treatment, and not replace other therapies such as avoidance of soap, regular and liberal use of moisturizers, and short bursts of topical steroids as needed.

Chapter 11
Allergy tests and eczema

One of the most common questions that people with eczema ask is whether they are allergic to something, and whether allergy tests may be useful. This chapter will help you understand what allergy is all about, and how it can relate to your eczema. Although allergy tests do not always provide a simple answer to the cause of your eczema, they can help identify important triggers in some people. This chapter looks at the different forms of allergy tests available and discusses when they are likely to be helpful for you as an individual.

What is an allergy?

Before discussing allergy tests we need to understand what an 'allergy' is (see Box 1). In simple terms, an allergy is an overreaction of your body's immune system to something that is normally harmless. Your body's immune system, which is designed to fight infections, is made up of many different types of cells in your bloodstream and in your skin. These cells produce proteins called antibodies, as well as many different chemicals (including histamine) every time infections get into your body. Your immune system remembers each individual infection and reacts more quickly the next time around. Because of this you don't usually keep getting the same infection again and again – you become 'immune'.

Sometimes your immune system can start reacting to harmless things in the environment such as foods, animals and pollen. Why this happens is not fully understood. Your immune system remembers these harmless things in a similar way so that every time you come into contact with that substance you get symptoms – this is what is called an 'allergy'. The symptoms of allergy can be immediate (usually occurring within minutes) or delayed (occurring within days).

Box 1: Allergies

An **allergy** is an overreaction (hypersensitivity) of the body's immune system to a substance that would normally be considered harmless.

The substance causing the allergy is called an **allergen.** Allergens are usually proteins.

Immediate symptoms (usually develop within minutes)
- itchy skin swellings lasting a few hours ('hives' or urticaria)
- swellings under the skin (angioedema) – these often affect the eyelids, lips or tongue
- runny eyes and nose
- wheezing
- stomach pains, vomiting and diarrhoea.

Delayed symptoms (usually develop after hours to days)
- itchy, scaly eczema
- worsening of asthma.

Immediate and delayed allergies

Delayed-type allergies involve white blood cells called T-cells. These T-cells produce chemical signals when a person comes into contact with an allergen (see Box 1) in the environment, and these chemicals then cause skin inflammation. In the skin delayed-type allergies cause typical eczema (red scaly skin) Delayed-type skin allergies are often caused by substances such as perfumes, cosmetics or metals. **Immediate-type allergies** involve overproduction of an antibody called IgE, and in the skin they usually produce urticaria (hives) with itchy, raised wheals lasting a few hours. Immediate-type skin allergies are more often caused by foods, medicines, pollens or latex rubber. However, immediate and delayed allergies can overlap, and it is now known that many allergens that have been linked to causing eczema can cause immediate and delayed symptoms.

Q. What is actually happening in my skin when I react to something I am allergic to?

This depends on what you are allergic to and what your symptoms are. Different parts of your immune system are involved in producing immediate and delayed symptoms.

Immediate allergies involve an antibody called IgE which your body produces. IgE attaches on to cells in the skin called mast cells. When you come into contact with something you are allergic to it gets into your skin and attaches on to the IgE antibodies which are stuck on your mast cells. This makes the mast cells release chemicals such as histamine into the skin. Histamine causes urticaria (hives) and itching.

Delayed allergies involve white blood cells called T-cells. These T-cells circulate in your blood and enter the skin. When you come into contact with something you are allergic to the T-cells recognize it. This makes the T-cells produce chemicals which cause skin inflammation and itching.

Q. Can allergies cause any serious symptoms?

Yes. Anaphylaxis is a rare form of life-threatening immediate-type allergy with severe swelling of the mouth or throat and difficulty breathing. Anaphylaxis can occur in people with or without eczema, but is more common in people with atopy (see Box 2). Children or adults with a history of anaphylaxis should ideally be seen by a specialist allergy team to ensure that they know exactly what to do in the event of a reaction. A self-injectable device containing adrenaline (also called epinephrine) may be prescribed for use in severe reactions – this will help counteract some of the symptoms but urgent medical attention is absolutely essential.

The role of allergy in eczema

Allergies can play a role in eczema but they do not seem to be the only cause of the condition in most people. Allergic contact dermatitis is the only type of eczema in which an identified allergy is the main cause of the condition. In people with atopic eczema, specific identifiable allergies can sometimes play a role but are rarely the main cause; many different things usually play a role (see Chapter 2). This is why people with atopic eczema may

Box 2: What is anaphylaxis?

Anaphylaxis is a sudden, serious allergic reaction, which occurs when the body reacts abnormally to a harmless substance such as peanuts, other foods, insect bites, latex or medicines.

What are the symptoms?

The symptoms of anaphylaxis are:

- sudden difficulty in breathing
- severe asthma
- swelling of the throat and mouth
- difficulty in swallowing or speaking
- alterations in heart rate
- generalized flushing of the skin
- nettle rash (hives) anywhere on the body
- abdominal pain, nausea and vomiting
- sense of impending doom
- sudden feeling of weakness (drop in blood pressure)
- collapse and unconsciousness.

The respiratory (breathing) symptoms are the most common. It is worth bearing in mind that not all individuals necessarily have all the symptoms.

Severe symptoms

The most severe symptoms of anaphylaxis are:

- swelling of mouth, lips or tongue which cause difficulty swallowing and talking
- sudden difficulty in breathing
- fainting or collapse.

These symptoms require immediate treatment. If you are believed to be at risk of having a severe reaction you will have been prescribed an EpiPen® by your specialist team. If you have to use your EpiPen® or you have a severe reaction someone must dial 999 for an ambulance and tell the staff that you are having an **anaphylactic** (pronounced anna-fil-actic) **reaction**.

contd.

Mild allergy symptoms
Some people find that the allergy symptoms they experience are always mild:

- redness around the eyes
- lip swelling
- slightly puffy face
- red blotchy rash on face or hands
- stomach ache
- nausea
- irritability
- tickly throat/tingly tongue.

If mild symptoms develop and your doctor has given you an antihistamine medicine, take it straight away and keep a close eye on your symptoms in case they develop into more severe ones.
For further information contact the Allergy UK and Anaphylaxis Campaign (see Resources for details).

---

sometimes improve with allergen avoidance but their eczema will not usually clear up completely. Different allergies affect people with eczema differently, and working out what affects you as an individual is not always easy. Some types of eczema are not thought to be primarily caused by allergies, for example, seborrhoeic eczema, irritant contact eczema and gravitational eczema.

Q. Which type of allergy is more significant as a cause of eczema – immediate or delayed?

This depends on the type of eczema you have, as both immediate and delayed allergies can play a role. The allergens that have been most closely linked with atopic eczema (such as house dust mites, pollen and foods) usually produce immediate allergic symptoms, but they may go on to produce delayed symptoms with time (for example, worsening of your eczema). Allergic contact dermatitis (see Chapter 1) is caused by a delayed allergy to something coming into contact with the skin. Pompholyx eczema may sometimes be caused by immediate or delayed allergies.

Allergy tests in eczema

Allergy-testing can be used *as a guide* to whether you are allergic to something or not, but it is important to understand that allergy tests are not perfect. This means that a positive test is not always proof that you have an allergy, nor that the allergy is making your eczema worse.

Allergy tests are not needed in everyone with eczema. They are most helpful in people whose symptoms strongly suggest that allergy may be contributing to their eczema. Allergy-testing may also be used if your eczema is not getting better with simple treatments. It is important that whoever is doing the investigations is experienced in performing allergy tests *and* interpreting the results in the context of your symptoms.

Q. What allergy tests are available on the NHS for people with eczema?

There are three main types of allergy test: blood tests, skin-prick tests and patch tests. Blood tests and skin-prick tests look for immediate-type allergy, and patch tests look for delayed-type allergy. Sometimes more than one test needs to be carried out to help work out what you are allergic to.

Blood tests for specific IgE

As mentioned earlier, in immediate allergies your body makes increased amounts of an antibody called immunoglobulin E (IgE for short) against whatever you are allergic to. The level of these antibodies in the blood can indicate what your body might be overreacting to. The test is straightforward to perform and involves a single blood sample which can be used to test for several different allergies. However, the result may take many days to come back. In young children a cream can be put on to numb the skin 30 to 60 minutes before the blood test if necessary.

Skin-prick tests

These tests are similar to blood IgE tests as they are used to look for immediate-type allergies to common substances in the environment (see below). A small drop of liquid containing each substance to be tested is put on your skin (usually your arm). A tiny scratch is made through each drop so that the liquid can get through the top layers of your skin. If you are allergic to something a small swelling (called a wheal) develops around the scratch, usually within 15 minutes. The tests do not usually hurt very much at all.

Patch-testing

This type of allergy test is used to look for delayed-type allergy to things coming directly into contact with the skin (allergic contact dermatitis – see Chapter 1). Standard patch tests are not used to test for food allergy or other immediate allergies. If you have atopic eczema, patch tests may be used to see if a contact allergy is making your eczema worse. Your back needs to be fairly clear of eczema to have the tests performed. Several small round aluminium discs (usually 30 or more) are stuck on your back with sticky tape strips for two days. Each disc contains a different substance that is being tested. The patch test nurse will put small pen marks around the tape, which mark the position of each disc. When the patches are removed after two days, you can have a bath or shower. You need to go back to the hospital two days after the patches are removed for the doctor to examine your back. If you are allergic to any of the substances in the discs, a red inflamed patch of skin that looks like eczema will have developed under the disc.

A special form of patch-testing called the atopy patch test has recently been developed. In the atopy patch test substances that usually cause immediate symptoms (for example, pollens, house dust mite and foods) are applied to the skin in a similar way to standard patch tests, to see if they cause a patch of eczema. In the future the atopy patch test may provide a better guide to whether foods and substances in the air like pollens could make eczema worse, although as yet the test is still experimental and not widely available.

Q. Who should I see to discuss allergy-testing for my eczema?

You should first see your GP, who can refer you on appropriately. Many different specialists do allergy tests in children and adults with eczema, and exactly who you see will depend on the services in your area. Some experienced GPs with a special interest in eczema will carry out allergy tests. However, more often your GP will refer you to your local dermatologist (skin doctor), paediatrician (children's doctor) or immunologist (allergy doctor), depending on what type of allergy test you need. Although blood tests can be carried out anywhere, skin-prick tests and patch tests require special facilities and are usually carried out in a hospital. Skin-prick tests are usually carried out by allergy doctors working in special allergy clinics. Patch tests are usually carried out by dermatologists working in a skin department.

Q. I have seen a number of allergy tests advertised in magazines and on the Internet. Should I have one of these tests instead of waiting for my GP to refer me for allergy-testing on the NHS?

An increasing number of allergy tests are now being advertised in private clinics by alternative practitioners working outside the NHS. Some of these tests are based on blood IgE levels, although the quality of the tests can vary greatly and it is impossible to give any guarantee that they will help your eczema. Many of the tests are expensive. In the case of some alternative forms of allergy-testing there is absolutely no proof that they give accurate results in patients with eczema. These unproven forms of allergy-testing include applied kinesiology, hair analysis and VEGA testing.

Applied kinesiology is a form of allergy-testing which claims to be able to detect allergies and intolerances to substances such as foods and drugs using kinesiology (the study of movement). The test involves a practitioner moving various parts of your body (usually the shoulder) to detect changes in muscle strength, which are claimed to reflect disturbances in the body's energy fields caused by particular allergies. Applied kinesiology is of no proven practical use in people with eczema.

Hair analysis involves sending hairs (usually from the back of your head) to practitioners who measure the levels of various minerals and vitamins in them. The levels of these substances in the hair can be significantly affected by many unrelated factors, and there is no evidence that they relate to allergy or eczema in any way.

VEGA (or electrodermal) testing involves measuring the electromagnetic conductivity of the human body. An electrode is attached to an acupuncture point (often the toe) and the patient holds a second electrode, while the allergens to be tested are placed in a honeycomb chamber in the circuit. Changes in conductance are measured using a galvanometer and low readings are taken to indicate allergy or intolerance. There is no medical evidence that VEGA tests have any diagnostic accuracy in the management of eczema.

Q. Could conventional allergy-testing have any side-effects or make my eczema flare up?

Blood tests have no risk of side-effects as they don't involve you coming into contact with any allergens.

Skin-prick tests can cause itchy wheals on your skin but these settle very quickly. Very occasionally skin-prick tests can trigger a severe allergic reaction (anaphylaxis). This is most likely with severe food allergy (especially peanuts) or latex allergy. For this reason skin-prick tests should always be performed where resuscitation facilities are available. It is unlikely that skin-prick testing will trigger an eczema flare-up, but this is possible. Antihistamines need to be stopped at least 48 hours before skin-prick testing as they can interfere with the results, so if you also suffer from hayfever this may temporarily become worse.

Patch-testing can make some people's backs itchy and uncomfortable. Some people with atopic eczema develop a flare-up of their eczema under all the patches (angry back) which makes it difficult to read the results. There is little risk of triggering anaphylaxis as patch tests are used to investigate allergens that tend to cause delayed symptoms.

Q. Can allergy tests be carried out in children?

Yes, they can if they are felt necessary. However, young children don't like having blood tests taken, and may not co-operate with skin-prick testing. Patch-testing is time-consuming and unfortunately children often pull the patches off, which makes it impossible to get a true reading.

Q. What allergies can be tested for?

Blood tests and skin-prick tests are most commonly used to look for allergies to:

- foods – more than 150 different foods can be tested for, although the most common foods to cause immediate allergy are milk, eggs, peanuts, tree nuts (for example, brazil nuts and almonds), wheat, fish, shellfish and soya
- latex rubber
- grass and tree pollens
- house dust mite.

Patch tests are most commonly used to look for allergies to:

- perfumes and fragrances
- metals in jewellery
- cosmetics and toiletries
- antibiotic creams
- steroid creams
- preservatives in creams and moisturizers
- Elastoplast and adhesive tapes
- lanolin
- glues and resins
- cement
- plants
- rubber
- hair dyes
- local anaesthetics.

Q. If I have a positive allergy test does it mean that I am definitely allergic to that substance?

Not necessarily. Patients with atopic eczema often have high levels of IgE antibodies in the blood anyway, so a positive blood test or skin-prick test is not always proof of allergy. It is common for people with atopic eczema to show many positive results with blood and skin-prick tests even when they are not allergic to the substance being tested, so the result always needs to be interpreted carefully by an expert in the context of your history. A positive allergy test along with a history of typical allergic symptoms makes it more likely that you are allergic to that substance.

Q. Does a positive allergy test mean that the allergy is making my eczema worse?

Again, not necessarily. High IgE levels can occur as a result of other allergic diseases that you may be suffering from such as asthma or hayfever, and may have nothing to do with what is happening in your skin. For example, if you get hayfever each spring and summer but your eczema gets better in the pollen season, a positive skin-prick or blood test to pollen is more relevant to your hayfever than to your skin. A positive blood test or skin-prick test to something does not always mean that your eczema will improve by avoiding the substance. Some people show positive patch test results to substances that are causing them no problems in day-to-day life. The symptoms you have had in the past are significant in deciding whether the allergy test result is relevant to you as an individual.

Q. Is food allergy a common cause of eczema?

Although food allergy may play a role in atopic eczema, foods are not thought to play a significant role in other types of eczema. Overall, food allergy is not thought to be a common cause of atopic eczema but it may be an important factor in a small number of patients. Food allergy is most likely to be important in children under the age of three whose eczema does not respond to simple treatment. Food allergy and atopic eczema can occur separately: not everyone with food allergy has atopic eczema, and not everyone with atopic eczema has food allergy. However, people with atopy (atopic eczema, asthma or hayfever) are more likely to develop food allergies than people who are not atopic. In some people food allergies just produce immediate symptoms such as urticaria (hives) in the skin. In others certain foods may cause or worsen their eczema if the food continues to be eaten on a regular basis. The eight most common foods to be allergic to are milk, eggs, peanuts, tree nuts (for example brazil nuts and almonds), wheat, fish, shellfish and soya.

Q. Should I put my child on a diet to see if food allergy is causing his eczema?

No. It is important to remember that cutting foods out of your child's diet will put extra stress on him and the family, and will make his life more miserable. There is also a significant risk that he will become deficient in nutrients and this could affect his growth and development. If your child's eczema is not clearing with simple treatment and you strongly suspect that certain foods are making it worse you should discuss the problem with your GP, who can refer you to the hospital for allergy-testing if necessary. Diets should always be supervised by a qualified dietician who can ensure that your child is following the diet properly and safely while monitoring his eczema.

Q. Does a positive allergy test to food mean that my child's eczema will get better if I cut the food out of her diet?

Not necessarily. Allergy tests give information on how likely it is that your child is allergic to a food, but they can't tell you for sure whether that food is or isn't making her eczema worse. If your child has symptoms of immediate-type allergy (such as hives or lip swelling) every time she eats that food, you should avoid the food to reduce the chance of her getting a more severe immediate allergic reaction (see Box 2 on page 135), and discuss the problem with your doctor and dietician. Avoiding the food in question may improve her underlying eczema but it doesn't always help. Keep a record of her symptoms over a six- to eight-week period after cutting the food out of her diet to see whether it has any long-term effect on her skin. Your dietician can help you with this.

Q. Does a negative allergy test exclude food as a cause of my child's eczema?

No. A negative blood test or skin-prick test means that it is very unlikely (but not impossible) that your child has an *immediate* allergy to that food. However, eczema can sometimes be caused by allergic mechanisms that don't involve overproduction of IgE and these reactions aren't detected by blood or skin-prick tests. Eczema can also be caused by reactions to food that don't involve true allergy – this is called food intolerance, and it is not detected by allergy-testing.

Q. What is food intolerance?

Food intolerance is a reaction to a food that does not involve the immune system, and therefore cannot be detected by allergy tests. It may be caused by low levels of enzymes in the gut that digest the food, and is sometimes inherited. If you are allergic to a food you are likely to react to even small amounts of the food. In contrast, symptoms of food intolerance are related to the amount of the food eaten, and often much larger amounts of the food can be eaten before symptoms develop.

Q. What are the symptoms of food intolerance?

The symptoms of food intolerance include abdominal pains, bloating and colic, but not immediate symptoms such as urticaria (hives). Babies and young children with food intolerance may show poor growth and failure to thrive. Some children and adults with food intolerance develop eczema which seems to improve when the food is cut out of their diet. If you think you have symptoms of food intolerance then discuss this with your doctor, who can refer you to a dietician.

Q. Can I tell if a food is making my eczema worse without having any allergy tests?

Yes. The best way to test whether a food is really making your eczema worse is to avoid the suspected food for four to six weeks and keep a diary of your eczema symptoms to see if your eczema gets better. This is best supervised by a dietician. If you avoid the food only for a few days it will be difficult to draw any conclusions because atopic eczema can fluctuate from day to day anyway, and flare-ups can take a few days to fully develop. You can then reintroduce the food slowly and see if it makes your eczema worse. It is important to cut out only one food at a time. As mentioned earlier, it is absolutely essential not to cut out foods from young children's diets without consulting your health visitor or doctor as growing infants may become deficient in nutrients. A dietician's input is essential in children and infants, especially if a staple food such as a dairy product is to be avoided. It is also advisable for a dietician to be involved in adults if significant dietary changes are involved.

Q. My baby's eczema developed when I started bottlefeeding him. Could he be allergic to cow's milk?

It is very common for eczema to develop during the first year of life and parents often worry in case it is caused by the introduction of cow's milk or certain foods. If your baby is otherwise healthy and gaining weight with no symptoms of diarrhoea, urticaria or lip swelling, cow's milk allergy is unlikely. Similarly, if your baby's eczema is mild and clears quickly with simple moisturizers and mild steroid creams, cow's milk allergy is unlikely. However, if your child is getting frequent diarrhoea and is often colicky and irritable after bottlefeeds or not gaining weight, he may have cow's milk allergy or cow's milk intolerance. In this case allergy tests (usually blood tests) may be helpful. In some hospitals doctors and dieticians prefer to eliminate cow's milk from the diet and then reintroduce it in a supervised manner ('milk challenge') once the baby's symptoms are under control, with close monitoring for any deterioration in his or her skin or other symptoms. If allergy tests or cow's milk challenge are positive, your doctor or dietician may recommend a low-allergy form of cow's milk formula (hydrolysed formula) until your child has outgrown his allergy. If allergy tests are negative, a trial of low-allergy formula milk is still sometimes recommended, depending on your baby's symptoms. Soya milk can also be tried in children over the age of six months, but over a fifth of people with cow's milk allergy or intolerance also have problems with soya milk.

Q. My five-month old baby has mild eczema. Should I change from cow's milk formula to soya milk just in case she is allergic to cow's milk?

Soya milk is not currently recommended before the age of six months as it contains small amounts of plant oestrogens called phytoestrogens (hormones) that could potentially affect your baby's development. It is also possible to become allergic to soya milk, just like cow's milk. If your baby's eczema is mild and she has no other symptoms, soya milk is unlikely to be helpful, but discuss this with your health visitor or doctor.

Q. My child's eczema is usually very mild but every time she eats eggs she develops a raised, itchy rash like hives which lasts a few hours. This rash doesn't go away with her hydrocortisone. How should I treat her?

Your child's symptoms suggest she is allergic to egg (immediate allergy), and with such clear symptoms allergy tests (blood tests or skin-prick tests) may not be necessary – discuss this with your doctor. You would benefit from referral to a dietician, who can give you advice on egg avoidance and discuss when it is safe to try and reintroduce egg into her diet. Raw or undercooked eggs are more likely to cause symptoms than cooked egg. If your child accidentally eats egg and develops hives again, she should take an antihistamine tablet immediately as this should help the rash settle over a few hours. Your doctor can prescribe some antihistamine tablets to keep at home. Steroid creams will help her underlying eczema but will not treat urticaria (hives). If she develops more severe symptoms after accidental egg ingestion (see Box 2 on page 135) you must seek urgent medical attention (your GP or Accident and Emergency department).

Q. I have heard that if my child is allergic to egg he shouldn't have his MMR vaccine. Is this true?

A large amount of evidence shows that the MMR vaccine is as safe for children with egg allergy as for other children. The MMR vaccine does contain traces of hen's egg, but it can be given safely to over 99 per cent of children who are allergic to eggs. Tell your doctor or practice nurse that your child is allergic to eggs. If he gets only a mild rash after eating eggs there should be no problem in vaccinating him in the normal way. Children who have had a severe anaphylactic reaction to eggs in the past (for example, throat swelling, difficulty breathing or collapse) can be given the vaccine in a controlled environment; either as a day case in hospital or in the GP's surgery with close supervision. Discuss this with your GP so that any special arrangements can be made. Dislike of eggs or refusal to eat eggs is not a reason to withhold the vaccine from your child. Influenza (flu) and yellow fever vaccines can also contain egg and should not be given to people with egg allergy before consultation with a doctor.

Q. My one-year-old child has atopic eczema. Blood tests have shown that he is allergic to cow's milk and egg. Will he have to avoid these foods for ever?

No, he is likely to grow out of his allergies. Most children have outgrown cow's milk allergy by three years of age, and egg allergy by five years of age. Allergies to nuts and fish are the exception – these allergies usually persist into adulthood.

Q. Can allergies to food additives make eczema worse?

This is not thought to be common. Certain food additives (for example, colourings, preservatives and antioxidants) can release histamine from mast cells in the skin and cause urticaria, although they are not thought to be a major cause of eczema. Food additives which can cause urticaria include sulphites (in fruit juices, salads, wine and dried fruits), benzoic acid, parabens, antioxidants, flavour enhancers and colourings. These immediate-type food reactions cannot usually be detected by blood tests or skin-prick tests because IgE antibodies are rarely involved. Very occasionally food additives can cause a contact allergic dermatitis, either mainly affecting the mouth or sometimes a more generalized eczema. This is rare. The food additives implicated in allergic contact dermatitis include cinnamon flavouring (a flavouring in toothpaste, chewing gum, sweets and ice cream), sodium benzoate (a preservative in drinks, jams, jellies and other foods) and sorbic acid (preservative in foods such as cheese and syrup), among others. If your child is allergic to cow's milk he or she can react to casein (milk protein), which is often labelled as 'natural flavouring'. If you are concerned about food additives consider cutting them out for a trial period of four to six weeks; see your GP first to discuss whether you need to be referred to a dietician.

Q. My child often gets a red rash around the mouth immediately after eating fruit. Is this an allergy?

This is very common, and is often caused by an irritant effect of acidic fruit on the delicate skin around the mouth, causing redness and soreness, rather than a true allergy. However, some fruits (including kiwis, tomatoes, bananas, apples and plums) can cause an IgE-mediated urticaria on contact with the skin. Vegetables such as celery and onions can also cause IgE-mediated contact urticaria. Some fruits contain natural histamine-like substances called vaso-active amines which can cause redness and swelling of the skin without IgE being involved. Similarly, some fruit juice concentrates contain preservatives (sulphites) that can cause urticaria without IgE antibodies being involved.

There are some very simple measures which may help to prevent skin irritation caused by fruit. Try applying a layer of a greasy moisturizer (like Vaseline or Epaderm®) around the mouth before mealtimes; this protects the skin and can be gently washed off afterwards. You should then apply more emollient after patting the skin dry. If this fails, try cutting the food out of your child's diet for a few weeks before reintroducing a small amount into the diet again, and keep a record of his or her symptoms. If your child is getting severe urticaria around the mouth, or lip swelling, discuss the problem with your doctor as allergy tests may be needed.

Q. My child's eczema has been gradually getting better although she now has asthma. She recently went to a party and got swelling of her lips after eating some peanuts. What should I do?

Your child is likely to be allergic to peanuts, and you should see your GP to arrange allergy-testing to confirm this. In occasional cases where there is a strong suggestion of peanut allergy but allergy tests are negative, small amounts of peanut are given under close supervision in hospital. This is called a food challenge. Children who are allergic to peanuts do not always react to other nuts (for example, walnuts and brazil nuts). However, if your child is young your doctor is likely to advise avoiding all food containing nuts (peanuts *and* tree nuts) as labelling of food does not always distinguish between different nuts, and cross-contamination of nut products is common. Adolescents with peanut allergy (and no allergy to other nuts) can sometimes be safely educated to avoid peanuts and eat other nuts that they can tolerate, although this will very much depend on the advice from your doctor and dietician. Children and adults with nut allergy should have a supply of antihistamine tablets to take if they develop symptoms. They may also be given an EpiPen® to use if they develop severe symptoms, and a Medic Alert® bracelet to wear around their wrist (to alert others to the allergy if they become unwell). You should never be given an EpiPen® without being shown exactly how and when to use it. Unfortunately, most people with nut allergy don't grow out of their allergy, and therefore avoidance is usually life-long.

Q. I have heard that some creams contain peanut oil. Could these cause peanut allergy?

Some skin preparations including over-the-counter moisturizers do contain arachis oil (peanut oil). A few researchers have suggested that there may be a link between the use of these creams and the development of peanut allergy in some children. This may be because tiny residues of peanut protein are present in the creams. Research is still under way to resolve this issue, but meanwhile skin preparations and cosmetics known to contain arachis oil (peanut oil) are best avoided by families in which there is a history of allergy. Check the ingredients of any new products with your doctor or pharmacist before use.

Q. I work as a chef and keep getting red, itchy swellings on my fingers as soon as I handle fresh fruit and vegetables. Is this an allergy?

It sounds like you are getting contact urticaria. This is an immediate-type allergy which is common in food-handlers, and more common in people with a history of atopic diseases (for example, atopic eczema, asthma and hayfever). Foods known to cause contact urticaria include tomato, potato, garlic, celery, melon and kiwi, although several other foods can cause the condition. Many people notice the symptoms only on their hands, although it is possible to get itching and swelling of the lips or more widespread urticaria. Fresh food is more likely to cause contact urticaria than cooked or frozen food. The symptoms of contact urticaria usually settle within a few hours. Some people develop a protein contact dermatitis with repeated exposure to these foods. This looks more like a chronic hand eczema which flares up within half an hour of handling the food. Protein contact dermatitis involves both immediate and delayed allergy. In both contact urticaria and protein contact dermatitis it is the proteins in the foods that are responsible for stimulating the immune system and causing the symptoms. Wear plastic gloves when handling food as much as possible, and discuss skin-prick testing with your doctor. Antihistamine tablets are sometimes helpful.

Q. I get very itchy swollen hands within minutes of putting rubber gloves on. Could I be allergic to the gloves?

Immediate allergic symptoms after contact with rubber suggest latex allergy. Latex rubber is used to make a number of things, including rubber gloves, balloons and condoms. Any of these items can produce immediate allergic symptoms on contact with the skin (contact urticaria) if you are latex-allergic. Some people with latex allergy are also allergic to bananas, avocados, chestnuts, kiwis and other fruits – these foods contain a similar allergen to the protein found in latex rubber. It is important that you discuss your symptoms with your doctor, who can arrange blood or skin-prick tests to confirm latex allergy. Your allergy needs to be recorded on your hospital/GP and dental notes to alert clinical staff not to wear latex gloves if you require any medical procedures. Your doctor may recommend you wear a Medic Alert® bracelet. A wide range of non-latex gloves is now available; your doctor will provide you with more information.

Latex allergy almost always produces urticaria rather than eczema. If you develop itchy, scaly hand eczema (rather than immediate urticaria) a day or so after wearing rubber gloves, this is more likely to be caused by an allergic contact dermatitis to additives in the rubber such as thiuram. Discuss your symptoms with your GP, who can refer you for patch-testing if necessary.

Q. Skin-prick tests and blood tests have suggested I am allergic to house dust mite. Could this be making my atopic eczema worse?

Yes, it could. However, it is very common for people with eczema to have positive allergy tests to house dust mite, and unfortunately a positive allergy test does not always mean that your eczema will improve if you reduce the levels of house dust mite in your home. This is why allergy tests for house dust mite are not routinely performed in all people with atopic eczema. For some people, house dust mite levels affect their asthma more than their eczema. However, it is sensible to take the basic measures to keep house dust mite levels down in your home as much as possible (see Chapter 2 for details).

Q. How can I tell if I am allergic to my cat?

It is usually easy to tell if you have an immediate allergy to your cat as you will develop runny eyes, a stuffy nose and sometimes urticaria on your skin when you come into contact with the animal. It is more difficult to tell if your cat is actually making your eczema worse. If you notice that your eczema improves when you go away for holidays without your cat, you have some proof that cat allergy may be making your skin worse. Skin-prick tests and blood tests can give some guidance, so discuss allergy-testing with your doctor. See Chapter 2 for general advice on pets.

Q. My eczema always gets worse around my eyes each spring and summer. Could I be allergic to pollen?

Yes, you may be allergic to pollens, which are carried in the air and which can affect thin areas of delicate skin such as that around the eyes. Pollen can also get into the nose and airways and worsen hayfever and asthma. Skin-prick tests or blood tests can help identify what kind of pollen you are allergic to. Grass pollen may cause an itchy skin rash on your legs if you sit on the grass. People with pollen allergy can sometimes also react to fresh fruit and vegetables such as apple, cherry and celery (this is known as a cross-reaction) because the allergens have a similar chemical structure. In people who are allergic to birch pollen these foods may cause itching or swelling of the lips or mouth (oral allergy syndrome).

Q. What sort of people develop allergic contact dermatitis?

Anyone can get allergic contact dermatitis, from young children to adults. This type of eczema is caused by a delayed allergy to things coming into contact with your skin, and can be tested for by the use of patch tests (see above). Allergic contact dermatitis often occurs in people who have had no previous allergic problems. It can also can occur in people who already have atopic eczema; in this case you may notice your underlying eczema getting worse. People with atopic eczema do not seem to be at a particularly increased risk of developing allergic contact eczema, although they are more at risk of irritant contact eczema (see Chapter 1).

Q. I get very itchy, red areas of eczema on the front of my stomach every time I wear my jeans. I have also noticed that my ears get sore if I wear any jewellery that isn't gold or silver, and sometimes I get eczema under my watch. Am I allergic to something?

You are almost certainly allergic to nickel, which is a metal often found in jean studs, jewellery and watches. Nickel is the most common cause of allergic contact dermatitis. It is more common in girls, and often starts in the teenage years as a result of ear-piercing (with studs that aren't sterling silver or at least 18-carat gold) or wearing cheap metal jewellery. Once you have become allergic to nickel you are usually allergic to it for life, as with most other contact allergens. Nickel allergy is generally obvious from the distribution and timing of the eczema. Patch tests are not usually necessary to confirm the problem but they can be performed if there is any doubt about the cause of your symptoms, or if your eczema does not get better by avoiding metals.

Q. How can I avoid nickel?

It is difficult to avoid nickel completely because many metals (especially silver-coloured ones) contain it. Therefore it is found in many household objects such as scissors, coins, jewellery, press studs, zips, paperclips, key-rings and kitchen utensils. Many nickel-allergic people will develop eczema only if their skin is in contact with the metal for a prolonged period, or if their skin is broken or hot and sweaty (this lets the nickel get into the skin more easily). Avoid prolonged contact with jewellery that isn't silver or gold, and all other nickel objects as much as possible. Try painting jean studs or fasteners with clear varnish or lacquer to prevent your skin coming into direct contact with the metal.

Q. I have heard that nickel in the diet can cause eczema. Is this true?

Some studies have suggested that people with nickel allergy and hand eczema may find that their condition gets worse if they eat certain canned foods, or acidic foods that have been cooked in stainless steel saucepans; small traces of nickel are released into the food in these situations. Many foods naturally contain small amounts of nickel and avoiding traces of nickel in the diet altogether is very difficult. There is not yet enough evidence that nickel-free diets are beneficial to many people, but if you would like to pursue this further ask your doctor to refer you to a dietician.

Q. Why have I developed eczema on my face at the age of 30 when I have never had it before? Although I use make-up every day I am still using the same cosmetics that I have used for years with no problems.

Most people assume that they cannot become allergic to something that they have been using for years. This is not the case. Allergic contact dermatitis can develop after months or even (as in your case) years of uncomplicated exposure to a substance. The eyes are often the first area to be affected by cosmetic allergy as the skin is very thin and delicate. Anyone who is regularly applying creams or cosmetics to their face and develops persistent eczema should ideally be patch-tested to exclude an allergic contact dermatitis.

Q. My hands have become very sore and cracked since I started a hairdressing job. I did suffer from atopic eczema when I was younger but the condition had cleared up. Could I have become allergic to something at my work?

Your eczema has probably flared up because of skin irritation rather than true allergy. Jobs such as hairdressing and catering require regular handwashing and contact with soaps and detergents, all of which can irritate your skin and cause your eczema to recur in adult life. Pay extra attention to good hand care by avoiding direct contact with chemicals, drying your hands carefully after washing, and applying a regular moisturizer after each handwash and throughout the day. You can treat your eczema with regular moisturizers, along with a steroid cream from your doctor if necessary. If these simple measures fail it is possible that you have developed an allergy to one of the products at work such as hair dyes, perming solutions or even your rubber gloves. Your doctor can refer you to your local dermatology department for patch-testing.

Q. I have been using a hydrocortisone cream for months but recently it has been making my eczema worse. Could I be allergic to it?

There are two possibilities for your worsening eczema. One is simply that hydrocortisone is not strong enough to control your eczema and that you need short bursts of a more potent topical steroid. However, if you think the hydrocortisone is actually making your eczema redder and itchier after application, another possibility is that you have developed an allergic contact dermatitis to the cream. It is possible to become allergic to either the hydrocortisone itself or to one of the preservatives in the cream, although both types of allergy are uncommon. Discuss your symptoms with your GP, who can refer you to your local dermatology department for patch-testing.

Chapter 12
Nursery and school

For any child, starting nursery or school can be a huge milestone. Children with eczema and their parents often find there are extra hurdles to overcome. In general, children with eczema can lead a full and fun-packed nursery and school life. What is important is that your child's individual healthcare needs are planned for in advance, and that those involved in caring for your child are made aware of his or her eczema and what it involves. Parents often tell us that staff and teachers don't understand eczema and how it affects their child. Good communication and education is essential. Before your child starts a new nursery, playgroup or school always try to meet the staff and teachers to plan your child's care. This is a good opportunity to provide the staff with any eczema information they need to help care for your child more effectively. There are some excellent booklets, leaflets and information packs available from the National Eczema Society for children, parents and their teachers (see Resources).

The most important issues to share and discuss with those caring for/educating your child are listed below.

- Eczema is an itchy, inflammatory skin disease that is not infectious.
- Eczema fluctuates, and itching/scratching may be worse if the child gets very hot, upset or exposed to things that can trigger a flare-up.
- Children with eczema require regular moisturizers to prevent their skin from becoming dry.
- When the skin is very dry and cracked it may restrict normal playgroup or school activities such as holding a pencil or pen.
- Constant itching and scratching, combined with disturbed sleep, may mean that children with eczema are late for school, lack concentration and at times fall behind with their work.
- There may be times when children with eczema are away from

school for medical appointments because their eczema is particularly bad. Close liaison between the school and doctor/nurse are essential if this becomes a repeated problem.

- Teasing can sometimes be a problem. Your child may not want to go to school because he or she is called names or other children don't want to play with him or her because they think they may catch something. Again, close liaison between parent, child, school and medical team are essential. All schools and nurseries should have a bullying policy so don't try to sort the problem out on your own. Ask for help.
- Children with eczema are more susceptible to infections such as cold sores and impetigo.
- Each child is different and may have specific and individual care needs.

Nursery and playgroup

Q. My one-year-old sucks her thumb at nursery, and it always takes longer to heal because she has eczema. Would I be better off giving her a dummy?

The reason your daughter's thumb takes longer to heal is because of the constant irritation from wet saliva. Many children suck their thumb, and as she gets older she will stop when she is ready. The use of a dummy is not recommended as this could create further problems with wetness and dribbling around the mouth.

Q. There is an outbreak of chickenpox at my daughter's nursery. Should I keep her at home because she has atopic eczema but has not yet had chickenpox?

Providing your daughter's eczema is mild and well controlled on treatment, there is no specific need to keep her off nursery. If she has very bad eczema with lots of broken sore skin, it would be better if she didn't catch chickenpox until her skin is under control because she may get very sore and uncomfortable. In this case consider keeping her away from nursery until the outbreak has settled, and discuss more effective eczema treatments with your doctor. However, remember that it can take up to 20 days after infection for the spots and blisters to develop, so it is possible that she has already caught the virus. Most children in the

UK will catch chickenpox before the age of ten and become immune to the virus – this means that they don't catch it again. Generally it is better to catch chickenpox in childhood as it tends to be milder in children than in adults.

Children on immunosuppressant tablets such as steroids, ciclosporin and azathioprine should not be exposed to other children with chickenpox if they haven't had the illness before. This is because tablets that suppress the immune system will make it more difficult for the body to fight off normal infections, and the chickenpox could become very severe and widespread. If your child has had any steroid tablets in the last three months see your doctor immediately, as she may need a special injection to help fight the virus.

Q. My child does many messy activities at playgroup with paints, potato prints and flour. Although she loves playing, she always gets eczema on her hands and it seems to get worse after these activities. What can I do to help?

Water and dusty substances such as flour can irritate the skin if you suffer from eczema. Some people also develop itchy hives (contact urticaria) on their hands after handling certain fruit or vegetables such as potatoes, and this may be contributing to your child's problem. A greasy emollient or barrier cream should be applied to her hands before playing, with cotton mittens over the top to provide more protection if needed. After play her hands should be washed and dried carefully (preferably using an emollient soap substitute and not soap) and more emollient applied. Ask your doctor to give you an extra pump dispenser of emollient to keep at playgroup for regular use. Encourage your child to get into the habit of using an emollient on her hands regularly. The playgroup teachers can help and encourage her to use her emollient and this in itself can be turned into a fun activity. It is important that you let her join in with all the playgroup activities as much as possible and not restrict her unless her hands become very sore or infected.

Q. Should I keep my child off playgroup after he has had his routine immunizations in case his eczema flares up?

Providing your child's eczema is well controlled, there are no special precautions you need to take. Your GP or practice nurse will give you general advice about keeping an eye on his temperature for a few days, but you do not need to keep him away from playgroup unless he is feeling unwell. Children's paracetamol (for example, Calpol®) can be used if he develops a slight fever.

There is little evidence that immunizations are a common cause of eczema flare-ups. Although some children may find that their condition gets temporarily worse after vaccination, many more have no problems at all. If your child already has infected eczema, it is best to delay his immunizations until he has recovered. However, it is very important that your child does receive all their immunizations. Many nurseries and playgroups will not admit children unless they are fully immunized.

Q. My baby's eczema always seems to get worse when she is teething or has a cold. Is there anything I can ask the nursery staff to do when she is in day care?

Babies who are teething or have a runny nose as the result of a cold will simply make the problem worse by rubbing or smearing their face with nasal secretions and saliva. This can trigger a flare-up of their eczema by making the skin sore, red and irritated. The nursery staff will need to work hard to protect her skin and keep her clothing dry. Frequent changes of cotton bibs and the application of regular emollients will help to protect the skin around the face, mouth and neck, so take a pump dispenser of emollient into your child's nursery.

Q. My child is being potty-trained at the moment and I've noticed that his skin keeps getting red and sore around his waist. Why is this?

If your child has recently started using trainer pants or pull-up nappies, these may simply be a bit too tight. Any friction or pressure can cause sweating and irritation of the skin, so try a slightly different size or brand, along with regular emollients to any problem areas. Parents often find that nappies irritate their child's eczema, especially around the waistbands and top of legs. No single nappy is better than others and it is very much a case of trial and error to find one that suits your child.

School

Q. My daughter has eczema. Who are the most important people for me to speak to before she starts school?

When your child starts school she is likely to be in contact with many more adults than at nursery or playgroup. Try to meet your child's teachers, midday supervisors and school nurse to discuss the issues listed at the beginning of the chapter. If your child has any specific dietary requirements it is also important to speak to the catering staff.

Q. My son starts school after Easter and I am worried about the uniform as many clothes seem to irritate his skin. Do you have any advice?

Children find cotton clothing more comfortable so school uniforms can sometimes be a challenge. Allow time to shop – don't leave it to the last minute. If you find it difficult to find suitable soft clothes to fit in with the uniform code discuss the issue with the school as there may be some flexibility if you make them aware of your son's particular needs. Many of the larger supermarkets are expanding their range of clothing, and a wide range of mail-order products are also available to suit children with eczema. The National Eczema Society (see Resources) keeps an up-to-date list of cotton clothing companies and stockists.

Q. My daughter is going to infant school soon and I am worried how she will manage her eczema as I put on all her creams. What should I do to make the move easier for us both?

Most children with eczema will need to use their emollients at school. The school day is far too long to get away with applying them only before and after school unless her eczema is mild. Plan ahead. Although your daughter may be too young to do this by herself you can teach her to do small areas such as her hands with support. The earlier you get her involved in caring for her own skin the better. You need to ask the school who will be available to help her, and arrange a special place for applying the creams. She may prefer to have an emollient that comes in a pump dispenser as this is usually easier to use at school and prevents hands going in and out of pots (which can contaminate the cream with bacteria). If pots of creams have to be used, a wooden spatula or clean spoon should be used to take the cream out. Always ask your doctor to prescribe an extra tub of emollient so that you can leave one at school, and some small tubes for school/swimming/sports bags. Alternatively, you can fill your own smaller pots with emollient for her bags; some children like to decorate a special pot for school. Do not take your daughter's steroid creams to school as these need to be applied only once or twice a day. It is generally much better for you to apply the topical steroids at home instead, to avoid any confusion at school.

Q. During the summer my son's eczema gets worse if the school playing field has been mown. His eyes swell and he gets itchy lumps on his skin. Should I stop him playing games?
It sounds like your son may be allergic to grass pollen. This usually causes symptoms of immediate allergy (see Chapter 11) such as itchy watery eyes, a runny nose or urticaria (hives). The symptoms are worse on exposed skin. Your son may benefit from taking a non-sedating antihistamine tablet on the days he does outdoor sports activities. If he is getting symptoms on a more regular basis or suffers from hayfever, he may benefit from taking an antihistamine daily during the spring and summer months. If antihistamine tablets make him feel sleepy discuss this with your doctor or nurse as there are many different antihistamine preparations available. He should be encouraged to play sports but should apply his emollients before he goes out and wash his face when he comes in whenever possible. This will protect his skin from contact with the pollen and may prevent his eczema from flaring up.

Q. My daughter hates doing PE because of her eczema. What do you suggest?
If she is embarrassed about her skin, discuss the problem with her PE teacher. Schools will often allow children to wear leggings or track suits rather than shorts if there is a good reason. She may find her skin gets more itchy if she gets hot and sweaty, so access to a shower and a place to put on emollients after PE is important. Good communication with her teacher is essential.

Q. Since starting school my son has been doing lots of sport and his feet have started getting red and cracked on the soles. What shoes are best for him?

This is a fairly common problem, especially in children with atopic eczema, asthma or hayfever. The skin on the soles of the feet (especially under the big toes and on the balls of the feet) becomes red, scaly and cracked, and this can be painful. The condition is called juvenile plantar dermatosis, but other names include atopic winter feet or sweaty sock dermatitis. The problem is related to friction, and is usually worse in the winter and more common in boys. It tends to affect young children, and the problem usually sorts itself out spontaneously by late adolescence.

Synthetic shoes and trainers made of plastic, rubber, nylon or vinyl should be avoided as they make the feet very hot and sweaty if worn for long periods. This increases the friction on the skin as the foot moves up and down. Open sandals or bare feet are best at home, with light leather shoes for school. Above all else, it is important that the feet are kept dry and the footwear fits well so the sole of the foot is not sliding against the insole of the shoe. Using cork insoles and cotton socks will help to keep the feet dry and less sweaty. Emollients and occasionally topical steroids may be helpful. If the problem doesn't settle it is important to exclude other causes of redness and scaling of the feet such as athlete's foot (fungal infection – see Chapter 1) or less commonly a contact allergic dermatitis to footwear (usually affects the top of the foot rather than just the sole) – discuss this with your doctor.

Q. My son has had a recent flare-up of his eczema which the doctor said was because of infection. He had a course of antibiotics and I kept him off school. Would he have been OK to go to school?

If your son's eczema is weepy, with yellow crusting and open sores, it is sensible for him to stay off school for two or three days until the antibiotics have started to work. Many children feel generally unwell and their skin gets very sore when their eczema is infected, so it is difficult to concentrate on school work. There is also a small risk of infecting other children. However, once he is feeling more comfortable and his skin is starting to improve he should be fine to go to school. He should always finish the course of antibiotics but can take them at school; you will usually need to sign a consent form for the teacher to give them to him.

Q. My daughter's eczema is so bad that she often needs bandages. Can these be continued at school as they do really make a difference to her skin?

Bandages are used for a number of reasons and there are several different types available to treat eczema (see Chapter 8). Medicated bandages are often left in place for two days at a time. Some people also find wet wraps helpful in the daytime as well as at night. The bandages should be applied at home but the school does need to be made aware that you are using them and what they are for, as they will make your daughter look different. Some children like wearing bandages at school because it makes them feel special. Others find that they get teased and feel shy about wearing them. It is important that your daughter feels comfortable. If she gets embarrassed, adapt her treatments to fit in with school and stick to using the bandages overnight or at weekends. Remember that bandages are necessary only if your child hasn't responded to first-line treatments with emollients and topical steroids, so make sure her topical treatments are all being used optimally before you put pressure on her to wear them. Discuss this with your doctor, nurse or eczema team if necessary.

Q. I visited my son's new school this week and noticed that the classroom he will be in was very hot. I don't want to make a fuss or embarrass him but if he gets too hot he scratches a lot, which could make his eczema worse.

Your concern is understandable: if he gets very itchy and starts scratching a lot it may affect his concentration or interrupt the lesson. The staff and children in his class should be made aware of this and be advised not to say 'don't scratch', which will make him feel guilty, more uncomfortable and want to scratch more. He needs to adopt some simple measures to keep cool; having a cold drink at his desk or a cool cloth may help. He will also need somewhere where he can easily apply his emollient as this can have a soothing and cooling effect. You also need to consider where he sits in class, and ask whether he can have a desk away from direct sunlight or radiators which may make him too hot and itchy.

Q. Should I stop my daughter from doing certain activities at school because of her eczema? I don't want her to be singled out for being different.

Your daughter wants to settle in school and not be any different from her friends. That's why it's important that you prepare her and the school. There will be some activities in school which may irritate her skin and she may need extra consideration before she participates in them. Some parents find that sitting on the floor or hard school chairs irritates their child's skin, and this can be rectified by using a simple cotton sheet or towel to sit on. If your daughter is using glues and paints she may find that applying her emollient beforehand protects her skin. A pair of cotton gloves for messy play/activities may also help. Specific activities which may irritate her skin or require more planning to ensure she can participate in them include:

- art and pottery
- craft, design and technology
- home economics
- school trips
- work experience.

Discuss any individual concerns with her doctor/nurse and teacher as there are ways to work around most issues and allow her to enjoy a full range of normal school activities.

Q. My son is on a dairy-free diet and takes sandwiches in rather than having school dinners. What should I do as he wants to try school dinners?

You will need to discuss his special diet with the school. Most schools can make provisions for special diets but you will need to meet the staff to see what the procedures are in your area. If he has had any serious reactions to dairy products in the past and carries an EpiPen®, the school needs to have all the relevant measures in place in case he does have severe reactions (see Chapter 11). This requires close communication between you, your doctor/dermatology nurse, school nurse and all school staff.

Q. My son is very fussy about his food and now he is at school it is more difficult to make sure he is eating a balanced diet. Should I be giving him any extra supplements to help his eczema?

The use of food supplements for children who have eczema is not recommended. Children with eczema should have their weight and height monitored as part of their care. Their height and weight will also be checked by the health visitor/school nurse or eczema team. If a child is on a special diet because of his or her eczema or is found to need supplements, they will be recommended on an individual basis and the child will be monitored closely. You can always ask for general advice regarding your child's diet from your health visitor, school nurse, GP, practice nurse or eczema team.

Q. Head lice are a real problem at my daughter's school. Should I be careful when choosing a product to treat them because my daughter has eczema?

Head lice infestations should be treated using lotion or liquid formulations. Shampoos are too dilute to be effective. Alcoholic formulations are effective but can sting, so for young children and those who have eczema, aqueous (water-based) formulations are advised. Your local pharmacist will be able to guide you.

Q. Since starting school my son's eczema has been terrible. What am I doing wrong?

Many factors may have contributed to your son's flare-up. Have a talk with him to find out if there is anything upsetting him at school. Has he settled or is he getting teased and being called names? Is he managing to apply his emollients when needed? Is the classroom environment comfortable for his skin? If you didn't originally visit the school it is worth arranging a meeting to discuss the issues and address any concerns. Also discuss the problem with your doctor and make sure there is no medical reason for his flare-up such as secondary infection. Do not feel you are to blame – sometimes eczema can go up and down without any reason, and your child may simply require a period of time to settle and adjust to school.

Q. My teenage daughter is going on a school trip. She is really worried about using her creams in front of her friends. Is there anything I can do to help?

Teenage years can be difficult, so do try to talk to your daughter about her concerns and worries. She will need to use her treatments when she is away or her eczema may flare up and ruin the trip. By this age she should already be taking responsibility for her skin care but she should also feel that she can ask you for help if she needs it. It's important she finds the creams and ointments acceptable. Often older children don't like the heavier greasy emollients or huge tubs to carry round. They like to be the same as their friends, so for the purpose of the trip she may prefer to use different emollients from those used in the privacy of home. Several products are available, and she may like to try a few out before the trip to find the one she prefers. All the emollients are available over the counter and once she has found one she likes, you could discuss this with your eczema nurse or doctor who can then put the product on prescription. Other anxieties she may have need to be considered. Will she have time to shower/bathe and apply her creams in privacy? If she will be sharing sleeping accommodation this may be worrying her. If your daughter is happy for you to discuss these matters further, arrange a private meeting with the teacher responsible. Often, good communication and simple planning can ease any worries considerably.

Q. My daughter is doing her exams at the moment and her eczema has started to flare up. How can I help?

Stressful exams are often associated with a temporary eczema flare-up. This is usually difficult to avoid completely, but the eczema tends to settle quickly when the stress is over. As exams are often held over the summer, heat and sweating can exacerbate the problem even further. Help her find a cool shady place to do her studies, and suggest she uses a lighter emollient in hot weather. It may be that she has neglected her treatment slightly while she has been under pressure from her work, and some gentle reminders are often all that's needed. Try to give her lots of positive encouragement and support, and make sure she is eating and sleeping well to keep her energy levels up and stress levels down. Avoid antihistamines as even the newer non-sedating tablets may reduce her concentration levels. If her skin flares up badly she may need some stronger eczema treatment to tide her over exam time – discuss this with her doctor or nurse.

Q. I will be choosing my options for GCSE and A-levels soon. I am not sure what career I want yet but are there any things I should consider given that I have eczema?

Most people who suffer from eczema are as capable as the next person in achieving their desired careers. However, if you have suffered from atopic eczema in childhood there are a few areas of work which could give rise to problems in later life, even if your eczema looks like it has cleared up before you leave school. These are mainly jobs involving 'wet work', which run the risk of triggering hand eczema. They include the following.

- **Hairdressing**: The frequent immersion of your hands in hot soapy water and the handling of hair colours, bleaches, perming solutions and other chemicals can all irritate the skin.
- **Catering**: The need for frequent handwashing and cleaning of utensils in hot water and detergents can irritate the skin. Regular contact with raw fruit and vegetables can also cause skin irritation or contact urticaria.
- **Engineering and motor vehicle repair**: This can involve almost continuous contact with oils and coolants, which can be extremely irritating, and occasionally cause an allergic contact dermatitis.
- **Nursing**: This profession involves frequent handwashing and regular contact with a variety of irritants. In addition, you run the risk of cross-infection between yourself and the patients or vice versa if you have active eczema. There are many areas within nursing where it would be possible for a person with eczema to work, but if you have a tendency to hand eczema, this could pose problems during training.
- **Animal handling**: Exposure to animal dander and fur can cause problems, as can the need for regular handwashing.

- **Plastering and bricklaying**: Contact with wet cement and dusts can irritate the skin. The chromate in cement can cause allergic contact dermatitis.
- **Work with adhesives**: Glues and epoxy resins can irritate the skin or cause an allergic contact dermatitis.

If you have set your heart on a career there are usually ways of minimizing the potential problems. Careful thought at this stage of your life can save a lot of heartache later. Your final career choice is a very individual decision and will depend on how severe your eczema is and which body sites are involved. Talk to your family doctor, nurse and school careers team.

Chapter 13
Social life and leisure

Eczema can affect many different areas of your everyday life, including social activities, sports and holidays. So how can you get on and enjoy your life, your family and friends as much as possible, without always being limited by your skin condition? This chapter gives you advice on how to make the most of your social life, leisure activities and holidays while still staying in control of your skin.

Sports

Q. My three-year-old daughter loves to go swimming but her eczema always flares up afterwards. How can I stop this from happening?

If your daughter enjoys swimming, encourage her to carry on, but remember that her skin is more susceptible to the drying effect of the water and chlorine. It is helpful to apply a layer of greasy emollient prior to swimming to protect her skin as much as possible. You don't need a really thick application or the emollient will just float off into the pool. After swimming, make sure she has a shower as soon as possible, then pat her dry gently and reapply her emollient. Don't be tempted to leave her shower until you get home, otherwise her skin will become dry and irritated very quickly. When using emollients in the pool be careful of slipping, and make sure you don't leave emollient around on the floor afterwards which could cause accidents. If there are several different swimming pools in your area, try different ones to find out which suits your daughter's skin. They don't all use chlorine and may use different methods to keep the water clean. If your daughter has a bad flare-up of her eczema or her skin gets infected, it is wise to avoid swimming until the flare-up has settled.

Q. My son plays lots of sports in his spare time. How can I protect his skin from further damage, especially when his eczema is bad?

All children with eczema should be encouraged to participate in as many activities as possible, so it is great that your son plays so much sport. However, he does need to be aware that various factors may make his eczema flare up or become irritated. Extremes of temperature and heavy sweating may well make him more itchy, so encourage him to wear thin layers of cotton clothes that he can take off during sports activities if he starts to overheat. A lot of sportswear is made of synthetic materials; avoid these if they rub or irritate his skin. If he is doing plenty of outdoor sport, remember that grass, mud and dust can all potentially make his skin flare up, especially on exposed areas such as the face, hands and legs. Applying an emollient before his sports activities will protect his skin and reduce the chance of eczema flare-ups. Washing or showering afterwards is important to remove any sweat and dust. If he has bad patches of eczema on his arms or legs, he could try a thin tubular bandage such as Tubigrip or Tubifast® on these areas during sporting activities, on top of his emollient or topical steroid. Try to find a regime that he finds easy; a comfortable compromise is sometimes necessary to keep the experience an enjoyable one for your son.

Q. My son wears shin pads for football twice a week. Although he's never had eczema before, over the last few weeks he's started to get very itchy and red under the shin pads. What should I do?

The most likely explanation is that he has developed patches of eczema owing to friction and rubbing from the shin pads, combined with irritation from heat and sweating. Although it is possible to develop a true contact allergic dermatitis to components of the shin pad itself this is extremely uncommon. Make sure he uses a regular emollient at least two or three times a day (from your GP or pharmacy), and see your GP if the symptoms don't settle after a few days as he may need a topical steroid to reduce the skin inflammation completely. If he needs to continue wearing the shin pads, use a layer of cotton bandage such as Tubigrip® or Tubifast® under the pads, over the top of his emollient. This will reduce the friction and help the emollient get into the skin effectively. See your GP if the problem persists despite these simple measures.

Holidays

Q. Our three-year old child has bad atopic eczema and we've always been worried about going on holiday in case his skin flares up. Have you got any tips about holidays in general?
Your concerns about holidays are understandable, although in fact most children's eczema improves when they are on holiday. Research has shown that many parents feel their choice of holiday is restricted because of their child's eczema, although with forward planning it is possible to find a good compromise that keeps the rest of the family happy too. Remember that holidays are for everyone and it's very important that you as parents also get time to enjoy a good break, otherwise the stress will rub off on to your child. You will need to think ahead about sleeping arrangements, climate changes, the need for creams, clothing, bedding and any special dietary requirements. Avoid old accommodation with thick carpets and curtains that can harbour plenty of house dust mites. Ask about air-conditioning and central heating if you plan to stay in a hotel – ideally you want to be able to adjust the temperature to keep the room cool at night. Take thin cotton sheets or a cotton sleeping-bag liner for your child's bed if necessary, and check that the beds don't have feather pillows and duvets; synthetic bedding is used in most holiday accommodation. Travel insurance and access to medical care is also important to consider, especially if travelling abroad. Ensure you plan well in advance and order adequate supplies of treatment from the doctor. If you need to carry pots of creams, bandages and extra medication check with the airline if your baggage allowance can be relaxed. If your child is on a special diet or allergic to foods make the airline aware. Many airline companies now have a nut-free policy but if your child does suffer from food allergies it is worth checking in advance. If you are going to a hot climate you may find that heavy, greasy ointments will be too occlusive, so consider lighter, cream-based products. Discuss this with your doctor or nurse.

Q. I am going on a sunny holiday to Spain. Will sunbathing help my eczema?

Most people will find that gentle sun exposure does improve their eczema, making it less red and itchy. This is why artificial light treatment is sometimes prescribed by dermatologists to treat patients with difficult eczema. However, too much sun can make you burn and increase your risk of developing skin cancer in the future. You need a safe balance. Allow your skin short periods of gentle sun exposure with suncream protection in the morning or late afternoon, but cover up with light cotton clothing at other times and avoid the strong midday sun (between around 11am and 3pm). A sun hat is a good way to protect the delicate skin of your face. It is very important not to get sunburnt as this will not only make your skin much more sore and irritated, but will also increase the risk of early skin wrinkles and skin cancer in the future.

Q. Which suncream is best for people who suffer from eczema?

Finding a suitable sunscreen or sun block is very much trial and error. What suits one person may not suit another. Ideally, find one which suits the whole family. For good sun protection use a sunscreen of at least SPF 15 (SPF 25 or more is recommended for children). Check the suncream label – it should protect against UVA (ultraviolet A radiation) and UVB (ultraviolet B radiation). Remember to reapply your sun protection regularly during the day, especially after swimming. If you are using other topical treatments for your eczema let them sink in completely before you put your suncream on (apply them at least 30 minutes before your sun protection if you can).

Q. Could suncreams make my eczema worse?

This is unlikely, although some people do find that certain suncream products irritate their skin. This is more likely if the product is fragranced. The best thing to do is try a small amount on a test area of your skin (for example, the inside of your arm) two or three times a day for two to three days to see if it irritates you. If you do develop a bad rash or flare-up of your eczema, try another product. If you find that you are having problems with many different suncreams, speak to your doctor, as very occasionally people become allergic to suncreams (allergic contact dermatitis). Some types of suncream allergy occur with application of the suncream alone. However, other types of suncream allergy are caused by an interaction between the suncream and the sunlight, so you get symptoms only when you have been out in the sun. This means that if you test the cream on an area of your skin overnight you may not notice any symptoms unless you then expose that area of skin to the sun. If you are worried about suncream allergy your GP can refer you for a special type of patch-testing called photopatch-testing in your local dermatology department.

Q. We recently went abroad and my son's skin seemed to flare up very quickly after the flight. Why did this happen?

The low humidity and the change of temperature created by air-conditioning in the plane may have affected your son's skin. It's always a good idea to take small pots of emollient on the plane to apply to exposed areas of skin during the journey. This will keep your son's skin moisturized and protected. Usually the flare-up will settle quickly after the flight.

Q. Should people with eczema avoid swimming in the sea?

No, not necessarily. In fact, many people find sea water very beneficial to their skin, and this is why some people use salt water baths to treat their eczema at home (see Chapter 10). However, salty water can sometimes sting and irritate the skin, especially if it is already inflamed and cracked. A good layer of greasy emollient applied before swimming will reduce the stinging. Ideally, have a shower as soon as you have been in the sea and reapply your emollient. This may not be possible on all beaches so find a compromise that suits your skin.

Q. What about swimming in the hotel pool?

This is no different from swimming in your local pool at home (see above). The chlorine or water additives can certainly dry the skin out, but a thin layer of emollient before swimming followed by a shower and more emollient should keep your skin protected.

Q. Will my eczema get better or worse on holiday?

Eczema is very individual and affects people in different ways, so it is difficult to predict accurately how your skin will behave on holiday. A combination of sun, relaxation and outdoor living will help most people's eczema enormously. However, others find that heat and sweating can make their eczema worse when they travel abroad. Part of learning to overcome your eczema is about becoming familiar with how your own skin behaves. So try not to restrict yourself, but learn what works best for you.

Growing up

Q. My daughter wants to go to her friend's house for a sleepover but I'm worried about her eczema flaring up. What should I do?

When children start school there will be many times when they want to stay away from home – this could be school or club trips, staying with family or sleepovers with friends. Sleepovers for the children are part of growing up. Children form close friendships at a very young age and this needs to be encouraged as much as possible. It's great that your daughter feels confident in the relationship with her friend. If she is happy to apply her treatments when she is away, this is an ideal opportunity to encourage her to become more independent in looking after her skin. If your daughter's eczema is severe, it may help to invite her friend home first so that she gets to see what living with eczema is all about. It is always better if you plan the night away when her eczema is as well controlled as possible and not during a flare-up. All children are tired after stopping over at a friend's anyway, and the added lack of sleep from scratching could make your daughter extremely miserable if her eczema is not controlled beforehand.

Q. I have just found out my daughter is trying to shave her legs. I am really worried that she may irritate her eczema. Should I tell her not to do it?

No, it's not usually a good idea to stop her from experimenting as she grows up. As soon as all her friends start shaving she is bound to want to try shaving her skin too – this is perfectly natural. However, her skin is going to be more susceptible to irritation, both from the friction of shaving itself and from any products used on the skin during shaving. Wet shaving can be done very effectively using the emollient she uses for washing, warm water, and a good-quality ladies' razor. The shaving should be done in a downward direction to prevent irritation of the hair follicles, which may result in itchy spots (folliculitis). By shaving in a downwards direction the hairs will be left slightly longer, but it will cause less irritation to the skin. Encourage her not to use blunt razors or soap-based products. After shaving she should get into the habit of applying her regular emollient. If her skin does get irritated she may need to use a topical steroid for a few days until things have settled. Other methods of hair removal such as waxing can potentially cause more skin irritation and are best avoided. Depilatory hair-removal creams are sometimes tolerated, but again can sting and flare the skin and occasionally cause a contact allergy.

Boys will also have concerns when they start to shave, and the same general principles apply. Avoid scented shaving foams/gels. If the skin gets irritated try using an emollient for shaving instead. Apply more emollient after shaving to soothe and protect the skin. After-shaves are best avoided if possible as they are often alcohol-based and can sting and dry out the skin. If after-shaves are used it is best to try a small test area for a day first before applying it to the rest of the face.

Q. My 11-year-old daughter wants her ears pierced. I am really scared it will make her eczema flare up but don't want her to be treated differently by her friends. Should I be firm with her and say no?

It is very much part of life that children and young people want to experiment with fashions and cosmetics. By saying no you will immediately create tension between the two of you, so try to find a compromise. It is important to remember the risk of contact allergy to nickel if she starts wearing cheap metal jewellery against her skin. Allergic contact dermatitis to nickel is a common problem that usually starts in teenage years and is often triggered by ear-piercing. If her eczema is well controlled, she is no more at risk of developing nickel allergy than her friends without eczema. However, if her skin is broken or cracked, the risk of developing nickel allergy does increase, as the nickel can enter the skin more easily and stimulate the body's immune system. If you decide that she can have her ears pierced, make sure the studs are British sterling silver or at least 18-carat gold, and advise her to avoid other metal jewellery including gold or silver-plated earrings as the coating can rub off very easily. Solid silver earrings (or 18-carat gold) are ideal, although they are more expensive.

Q. My daughter is going out a lot in the evenings with her friends and experimenting with their make-up. Is she best to avoid make-up altogether if she has eczema?

As much as possible allow your daughter to do all the things that other children of her age enjoy doing. You are right that certain cosmetics may irritate her skin given that she has eczema, but there is a wide range of products now available for sensitive skin which contain fewer additives and are less likely to cause a problem. Allow her to experiment a bit and learn what triggers her eczema and what doesn't. True allergic contact dermatitis to make-up can occur, but it is probably no more common in people with atopic eczema compared to those without. However, it is wise for her to use cosmetics labelled as 'hypoallergenic' if possible as these are less likely to cause contact allergy. If she has active eczema on the face, it is best to avoid all make-up and cosmetics and to stick to a simple light emollient. If she develops more severe eczema on her face, ask your doctor whether a mild topical steroid or topical immunomodulator is indicated (see Chapters 6 and 7).

Q. My son has got really bad acne on his face and back. How can he treat his acne without making his eczema worse?

This is a difficult problem, because first-line acne therapy usually involves topical treatments that can irritate and dry out the skin. Many acne products are alcohol-based and are particularly harsh on sensitive eczema skin. The most commonly used topical acne preparations are benzoyl peroxide, antibiotic solutions and vitamin A-related creams (retinoids). All of these treatments could trigger an eczema flare-up on his face and make it very red and scaly, even if he doesn't usually get eczema on his face. The first thing to do is discuss the problem with your doctor. If his acne is bad, the best course of treatment would probably be a course of low-dose antibiotics by mouth for three months or more, along with a light emollient for any facial eczema. If his acne is very bad and causing scarring, your doctor may refer him to your local dermatologist to consider treatment with a tablet called isotretinoin (trade name Roaccutane®). Isotretinoin is a drug related to vitamin A that is very effective in treating acne but one of the main side-effects is skin dryness; it also has other potential side-effects that your dermatologist will discuss with you in detail. If your dermatologist recommends isotretinoin, make sure that he or she is aware of your son's eczema – he may tolerate only a lower dose of isotretinoin, and will need to use plenty of regular emollient to counteract the dryness.

Another problem to consider is that many eczema treatments such as topical steroids, Protopic ointment® and greasy emollients can make acne worse when used on the face and back. Therefore treatment will need to be carefully balanced, depending on the severity of his eczema and acne. Try to find a compromise by sticking to a light emollient alone on his face and back whenever possible. A wide range of facial emollients labelled 'non-comedogenic' are now available from pharmacies – this means that they are especially designed not to block the skin pores and trigger acne. Try to find a preparation that suits your son's skin and doesn't cause irritation.

Q. My teenage daughter has started to dye her hair regularly. I am really worried her eczema may get worse. What should I do?

The same principles apply to hair colours and dyes as to other cosmetic products. You need to get a balance between letting your daughter have the freedom to experiment, while still staying on top of her skin condition. At this age she needs to start taking responsibility for her own skin and working out what she can and can't use without making her eczema flare up. She may have no problems at all with hair dyes, especially if they are used on an occasional basis. If she does find her scalp is getting more itchy or scaly, the most likely cause is simple irritation from the chemicals in the dye. This will normally settle down quickly over a day or two with a gentle shampoo and a short burst of a topical steroid scalp preparation if necessary. Allergic contact dermatitis (as opposed to irritation) from hair dyes is much less common. Contact allergy doesn't usually develop the first time the dye is used – it usually occurs after repeated use as it takes a while for your immune system to become sensitized to the dye. If your daughter develops very red and itchy skin shortly after using the dye, it is likely that she is allergic to it. In that case, the scalp itself will be itchy and sometimes very inflamed, but the redness and scaling will be more noticeable around the hairline (for example, forehead, ears, neck), where the skin is more delicate. See your doctor if this occurs to discuss referral for patch-testing.

Chapter 14
The impact of eczema on feelings, emotions and relationships

Eczema is often seen as a trivial condition which doesn't cause any long-term general health problems and often goes away by itself given time. While it is true that eczema is not life-threatening, the psychological and emotional effects of the condition on both the patient and the family should not be underestimated. It doesn't matter whether the eczema is localized to one area of the body or widespread, it can still have a major impact on the quality of one's life. This chapter looks at the many different ways eczema can affect your feelings, emotions and relationships, with advice on how to cope with the psychological effects of the disease in your everyday life.

Tiredness and exhaustion

Q. I feel completely exhausted trying to control my child's eczema. He is constantly waking up in the night scratching. How can I help him to sleep better at nights?

Tiredness is one of the major issues that parents and children have to deal with. All parents will have experienced lack of sleep with a new baby, although generally this is short-lived. Having a child with eczema who wakes at night can lead to a relentless succession of broken nights over weeks or months, leaving you and your child utterly exhausted and irritable. This naturally affects your ability to cope in the daytime, and what would usually be simple tasks turn into major ones as a result of tiredness. Studies have shown that on average one to two hours are interrupted each night when children's eczema is problematic. It is miserable to see your child waking up scratching and parents often feel frustrated, helpless and unable to see an end to the problem. Here are some practical tips to help you break the cycle of sleep loss in your family.

1. *Treat your child's underlying eczema more aggressively*. The fact that your child's eczema is itchy enough to wake him means that it is not well controlled at the moment. The itch and discomfort associated with eczema causes scratching, which in turn provokes more itching and the eczema gets worse. A vicious cycle is set up, known as the itch-scratch cycle. Even when the skin is not particularly red and bumpy the eczema may still be very itchy so always take your child seriously if he complains of itching or is constantly scratching. There is no doubt that treating your child's underlying eczema is the best way of reducing the itching and helping him sleep. Use plenty of moisturizers and do not be afraid to use short bursts of topical steroids as prescribed by your doctor. If these are not controlling your child's symptoms, see your GP to discuss stepping up to stronger treatments as discussed in the previous chapters. Remember that these stronger treatments are perfectly safe if used properly as recommended. In fact you are much more likely to cause your child harm by leaving his eczema uncontrolled than by stepping up to stronger treatments. A short course of a sedating antihistamine taken an hour or so before bed may help your child to settle at night, until his eczema is back under control. Early treatment of infections and avoidance of things that irritate the skin such as rough clothing and harsh soaps are all other useful ways of reducing itching.

2. *Protect your child's skin from scratching*. Always keep your child's fingernails short and clean to reduce the damage from scratching. Cotton mittens can be useful at night although some children tend to pull them off. In young babies cotton mittens can be attached to the clothing. Bandages (see Chapter 8) can be very useful, both to protect the skin from night-time scratching and rubbing, and to help topical treatments work effectively. Discuss this with your doctor or nurse.

3. *Create an environment which will reduce itching*. Wrapping your child up in a thick duvet in a centrally heated bedroom will make the itching far worse. Keep the bedroom cool by

opening the window in the daytime and turning the central heating down low at night. Plain cotton sheets are often better than a thick continental quilt, which can lead to overheating. Loose-fitting cotton pyjamas (or, for a girl, a light cotton nightie) are best for your child to sleep in. Try giving your child a bath about an hour before bedtime, followed by plenty of moisturizers to cool the skin. Remember not to apply too thick a layer of greasy moisturizer in the hope that it will last all night. If emollients are applied too thickly they often make the child hot and sweaty, which in turn lead to more scratching. Find an emollient which suits your needs. Try to avoid the common problem of letting your child climb into your bed. This may encourage an abnormal behaviour pattern whereby your child learns to gain from his eczema, and this can get you into a vicious cycle of disturbed nights. It is also likely that your bed will be warmer than your child's bed and this in itself may make him itch more. It is better to go to your child's room and give him the love and care that he needs and then be firm and leave him to fall asleep in his own bedroom.

Q. How can I help my child get off to sleep when he is always scratching his skin? He seems to be going to sleep later and later and is getting really tired and irritable in the daytime.

As discussed above, it is very important to make sure you are treating his eczema effectively. If he is scratching because his eczema is not controlled, you may need a short burst of stronger treatment. Active, poorly controlled eczema usually looks red, but it may also be bumpy, weeping, dry or scaly. If he is complaining of itching, it is a good sign that his eczema is not controlled, so see your doctor or nurse to discuss more effective treatments. Antihistamine tablets or syrup can be useful for five to seven days if his eczema has flared but should not be relied upon for regular use; it is much more important to treat the underlying eczema properly.

In some children scratching becomes a 'habit', even when their eczema is well controlled. In this situation it may not be the itch of eczema but other emotions (such as feeling anxious, stressed or uncomfortable) which trigger an automatic response to scratch. This habit often occurs at bedtime, when they are not preoccupied with normal daytime activities. Telling your child to stop scratching is not usually very helpful and often increases his anxiety, causing him to scratch more. Try to gently make him aware of his behaviour and give positive feedback when he stops. If he is not tired it may be wiser to allow him to stay up a little longer so he is more likely to fall asleep as soon as he gets into bed. Most scratching occurs in the 'twilight' zone between sleep and wakefulness.

General advice on how to get your child off to sleep includes taking him for a drive, giving him a cool bath and reading books, and you must choose whatever you feel is most effective and right for your family. Try to prevent your child falling asleep in the day as this will obviously affect his ability to sleep at night.

Q. What can I do when my child wakes crying and scratching because of her eczema?

Sometimes very little is needed apart from cuddling your child and adopting simple measures such as stroking her skin and leaving her to go back to sleep. Application of a light, cream-based moisturizer is also a useful way of cooling the skin – this can be kept in the fridge for extra cooling effect if your child finds this helpful. If she feels hot, remove some of the bed clothes. If she is visibly tearing at the skin, causing it to bleed, you need to protect that area with some form of bandaging (for example, wet wraps) and start treating her eczema more aggressively with stronger treatments over the next few days. Discuss this with your doctor if you have not already been prescribed stronger treatments for flare-ups. If your child refuses to accept any bandages or creams, you may be able to negotiate a reward system whereby she will be allowed to, say, watch her favourite video after she has co-operated with treatment. It is most important that you honour this agreement, otherwise you will lose her trust. Finally, you should bear in mind that many children without eczema are poor sleepers and your child's eczema may not necessarily be the reason why she wakes frequently. If there is no difference in your child's sleep pattern when her eczema is good, it is likely that other factors are contributing to her poor sleep pattern. Talk to your health visitor or school nurse as they may be able to help you with a sleep programme.

Guilt and depression

Q. At times I feel guilty about having a baby with eczema. Is this normal?

Parents often experience all sorts of feelings when their baby develops eczema, including anger, guilt, fear, anxiety, frustration and loss of control. Everybody wants their child to be perfect, and instinctively parents often blame themselves for any health problems that their children develop. Mothers in particular often look back at every aspect of their pregnancy or child's early life to look for things they might have done wrong, but this is really not helpful. As discussed in Chapter 2, there is no sure way of preventing your baby from developing eczema. If there was, clear health guidelines would be in place to prevent children from getting eczema. So try to avoid the temptation to analyse what you have done wrong or blame yourself, because you are not to blame. Try to channel your energies into learning more about your baby's eczema so that you can control his or her condition safely and effectively. Remember that most children will grow out of their eczema in childhood, and that if it is well controlled it is unlikely to have any long-term effects on their health or well-being.

Q. My two-month-old baby has really bad eczema and it's making me feel so depressed I just don't know what to do.

This is a common feeling, and caring for a young baby with eczema can have a huge effect on your emotions for many different reasons. The main piece of advice is not to bottle your feelings up. If you do, the problem is unlikely to go away quickly and may get worse. Your feelings are probably caused by a combination of factors: concern that your child is in discomfort, fear that you won't be able to control the disease, frustration, exhaustion and lack of sleep. If you are caring for other children at the same time, this will put you under even more pressure. If you are the mother, your hormone levels change dramatically after birth and this can add to the problem, making you more susceptible to depression. The first people to speak to are your health visitor and GP, who can give you the emotional and practical support you need, and also help you get your baby's eczema treated effectively. You may also benefit from talking to other parents of children with eczema; ask your GP or health visitor if there are any local support groups in your area. The National Eczema Society (see Resources) also provides excellent support. If you are struggling to get on top of your child's eczema with treatments prescribed by your GP, don't suffer in silence – ask your GP to refer you on to a skin specialist for further advice (see referral guidelines in Chapter 4). There are a wide number of very effective treatments available for eczema so it's just a case of getting access to the right advice and treatment when you need it.

Q. I feel guilty and sad when I go to mother-and-baby groups because my baby's skin is so red and sore. I want to keep going but find it harder each time, and always come away in tears. Will it get easier?

Babies with eczema often have redness and scaling of their faces which makes their skin condition particularly obvious. Because eczema is so common the vast majority of parents will be fully aware of what your baby's skin condition is and know that it is nothing to do with how you have been caring for your child. However, occasionally people are ignorant or insensitive about the condition and either stare or ignore you totally. Sometimes people ask intrusive questions such as 'Has your child been burnt?' or 'Has he got chickenpox?', implying you are a bad mother because of your child's appearance. Remember that people also react inappropriately because they feel awkward, uncomfortable or unsure as to how to react. All these situations will make you feel angry, guilty, upset and frustrated. Having the confidence to deal with these situations is not always easy. If you feel strong enough it does usually help to explain what eczema is rather than just ignoring the questions. Having another parent or someone who has been through the situation can also be very beneficial. Local support groups or the National Eczema Society and Changing Faces (see Resources) can help.

Anxiety and worry

Q. My son makes a mess of his skin when he scratches. I worry so much about the harm he is doing to himself and whether he is going to be left scarred.

There will be times when despite your best efforts your son will just have to scratch his skin. Fortunately, most scratches heal up really well over time and scarring is extremely unusual. Sometimes the skin can look a little darker or lighter where your child has scratched, especially if he has had poorly controlled eczema for some time. These dark or light patches can last for a few weeks or even months but will eventually fade. There are many ways of reducing the damage from scratching. The simplest way is to keep your son's nails well trimmed so that they are less likely to cut the skin when scratching. If your son tends to tear at his skin during the night when half-asleep, make it more difficult for him to get at his skin (for example, by making him wear a one-piece night suit). Bandages at night (such as wet wraps) are another way of giving his arms and legs a rest from the damaging effects of scratching but these should always be demonstrated by an experienced doctor or nurse.

Q. My ten-year-old child always scratches more when she is worried or upset. What can I do to help?

First of all make sure that her eczema is as well controlled as it can be. If she is upset, it can sometimes make her eczema worse; be prepared to increase her treatment if necessary to catch any flare-ups early. If your child's eczema looks clear but she is still scratching, it may be a nervous habit, and she is probably not aware that she is doing it. Talk to her and find out what is worrying her. If she continues to scratch, try these simple measures.

- Never say, 'Stop scratching!' All this does is make your child more anxious, which will make her want to scratch more when she is out of your sight. All advice needs to be positive and active.
- Give praise when there is no scratching.
- When your child feels the urge to scratch, teach her different ways of dealing with the itch such as clenching the fist tightly

for 30 seconds or pinching or tapping the skin where it itches. This takes the sensation of itch away without damaging the skin. This requires practice and a lot of encouragement.

- Use a reward system to praise your child for not scratching. For younger children it might be useful to use a star or sticker chart. You can either make a chart yourself, or buy a calendar with a space for each day on which your child could put the stars or stickers.
- Help her put her creams on at least 20 minutes before bedtime, to reduce irritation at night before she goes to sleep.

Q. I am really worried about using any steroid creams on my eczema in case they damage my skin. My eczema is really sore and itchy but I'm so frightened of damaging myself permanently with the steroids that I'm using only a moisturizer.

This is a very common worry among patients and parents and is one of the most common reasons for people to under-treat their eczema. In one study, three-quarters of parents of children with eczema attending the hospital clinic admitted to being worried about side-effects from topical steroids. Most parents worried about thinning of the skin (skin atrophy), although others were concerned about the effects of steroids on growth and development.

In the vast majority of patients there is actually very little risk of side-effects from topical steroids provided the treatments are used properly. You are much more likely to suffer harm by leaving the eczema untreated as this can lead to infection, exhaustion and a miserable quality of life. Under-treatment of eczema is a much bigger problem than over-treatment. When steroid creams were first introduced in the 1960s and 1970s there was much less knowledge about their use and safety compared to nowadays. Some people used strong preparations inappropriately for long periods of time, and this resulted in skin thinning and stretch marks. It is now extremely uncommon to see side-effects from topical steroids, even in people with severe eczema who have used their steroids intermittently for months or years. Many research studies have been carried out using ultrasound scans to monitor skin thickness during topical steroid treatment. These studies have suggested that the best and safest way to use topical steroids is in intermittent bursts, followed by steroid-free holidays until the eczema flares up again. The strength of topical steroid you will need depends on lots of factors such as your age, body site affected and thickness of your eczema. These issues are all discussed in detail in Chapter 6.

Your relationship with your GP and nurse is extremely important. Studies have shown that patients who are satisfied with the relationship they have with their doctor are more likely to understand and use their treatments, and have any fears allayed. Remember that some GPs have had limited training in skin-disease management; if necessary your GP will refer you to your local dermatologist to reassure you how you can use your topical steroids safely without the fear of side-effects.

Q. There is so much information on eczema, I feel I am sinking with it all. What should I do?

You may feel bombarded with information from family and friends, books and magazines, and on the Internet. The trick is to keep things simple. Concentrate on the basic skin care information your GP has given you first. If you still feel confused, ask to be referred to a skin specialist. Always ask your doctor or nurse for a written plan to give you a record of how to use your treatments; it is well recognized that most patients remember only a fraction of what is discussed in the consultation because of information overload. Everyone's eczema is different, and a good consultation is the best way to share your worries, clarify any confusion and tailor your treatment to you as an individual. The National Eczema Society is an excellent additional source of information and can provide telephone advice and support if you feel you are getting overwhelmed.

Irritability

Q. My job is very stressful, especially when I'm constantly itching. At the end of the day I always find myself snapping when I get home. Is this normal?

Living with eczema can put a strain on everything, including work and family life. If the stress builds up you may feel very low or anxious and have a short fuse. Everyone copes with stress and anxiety in different ways; it may mean taking up an activity to take your mind off the problem, or simply talking to a friend, your partner or a healthcare professional. It's certainly worth making sure you are treating your eczema as best you can (see previous chapters) as constant itching can really wear you down. Think about any triggers at work (see Chapter 2) and avoid these as much as you can.

Q. My son gets very upset and irritable when he has a bath. Is there a reason for this as he used to love bathing?

When children have a flare-up of their eczema or their skin is very dry they often complain of stinging in the bath or shower. If this is the case, let him go without a bath for a few days and apply regular moisturizers to repair the skin barrier before reintroducing bathing. Try out different emollients in the bath as some may be better tolerated than others – this is very individual.

Q. My child often gets cross and frustrated at the simplest of activities. Do you think this behaviour is related to his eczema in any way?

Parents of children with eczema often find that their children get cross and frustrated very quickly and don't concentrate for very long on a particular task such as reading or playing. As a result they are often described as 'naughty' children. However, parents commonly see a dramatic change in children's behaviour once their eczema is well controlled. Imagine trying to concentrate on a task when your skin is very itchy or you have had no sleep. Gaining good control does improve your child's ability to play and interact with others, so speak to your doctor about how you can control his skin more effectively if you think his eczema is active. Your health visitor or nurse can also be a useful source of advice regarding your child's behaviour in general.

Relationships

Q. I always want to ask my GP questions but don't always feel confident. I'm worried he may think my questions trivial.

Having a good relationship with your doctor or nurse is very important when you are learning to take control of a chronic condition such as eczema. Never feel that any question is too trivial – the more you ask the more in control of your skin you will become. Sometimes patients feel pressurized if the consultation time is short, and it is easy to forget what questions you wanted to ask. It helps to write down specific questions in a diary or journal beforehand to target your thoughts. Your doctor or nurse should find out what you and your family want to know and allow you the time to ask the questions.

Q. My doctor has been very supportive but I don't really feel he is able to give me all the information I need. How do I find out more about eczema?

Success in managing your eczema does not rely solely on applying creams. You need to develop an in-depth knowledge of your own skin, recognizing the pattern of eczema, how it responds to different treatments, and what triggers it to flare up. It is very difficult for your GP to provide you with all this information in a standard consultation, so other sources of specialist knowledge can be extremely useful. As well as the information provided in this book, a number of useful resources are listed at the end of the book and they can add to your knowledge even further.

Q. I have always suffered from bad eczema on my face and constantly feel that people are staring at me. Because of this I've started avoiding my friends and colleagues as much as possible, even though I want to be sociable and join in. Do you have any advice?

Eczema can have a significant impact on interpersonal relationships. If your self-esteem is low or you feel embarrassed about your skin, you may come across as very distant. This can make it hard for friends and colleagues to know you properly, even if you are longing for some close friendship. It can be difficult initially, but if you think positively and be open and friendly you will be surprised at how understanding your colleagues are. They may know very little about eczema, so explain a little about the condition and talk to them about your feelings rather than bottling them up. People will warm to you much more if you let them interact with you, rather than hiding away.

The other thing to consider is whether your eczema treatment can be improved in any way. Talk to your doctor about the safe use of topical steroids on the face, or discuss topical immuno-modulator therapy if steroids and emollients aren't controlling your skin. Think about any possible triggers such as pollen or cosmetics, and ask your GP about allergy-testing if necessary.

Q. My relationship with my husband has really suffered since our child was born with eczema. Is there anything I can do to help?

This is a very common problem. Caring for a child with eczema can result in lack of sleep, lack of time and general irritability, all of which can put a strain on relationships. Mothers often also find themselves being overprotective of the child with eczema, which can lead to feelings of jealously in partners as well as other family members. There are no right or wrong answers, but close communication is central to improving your relationship. Communication is usually the first thing to break down; you may be too busy to talk in the daytime and too tired at night. Try to put aside regular times to talk in the daytime before you get too tired. Don't bottle up your emotions because this will increase the tension between you both; explain how you are feeling. Your husband may like to get more involved in caring for your child if you have been doing a lot of the work. Not only will this improve his confidence and make him feel more part of the family, but it will take some of the strain off you and be extremely beneficial for your child.

It is important that you as parents try to find some time to relax. Studies have shown that parents of children with eczema are less likely to pursue leisure activities than other parents. Even if you feel tired and exhausted, taking up a leisure activity once or twice a week can help reduce stress levels enormously. Try to have some regular time together in a relaxed environment away from your child. This may mean getting a baby-sitter and going out for a drink or meal every now and again in the evenings.

If the relationship is still suffering despite your best efforts, you may benefit from some psychological support such as coun-selling. Discuss this with your husband, and speak to your GP if this is an avenue you would both like to pursue.

Q. When my son's eczema is bad, my daughter gets cross and angry with us. What can I do to help the situation as it is wearing me out?

It can be difficult juggling the demands of family life but do try to have some boundaries. Your daughter is probably feeling left out and jealous of the attention and time you spend with your son. Set limits for acceptable behaviour and also plan some time for your daughter so she doesn't always feel second best. Depending on her age you may be able to explain why your son needs to be looked after, and perhaps get her more involved – ask her to bring the creams or even help put them on your son. This can help her feel more important, and may increase the emotional bonding between your children.

Q. Only two of my four children have eczema, but all my time seems to be taken up applying their treatments. How will this affect my relationship with my other children in the long term?

Eczema can affect the whole family. However, studies have shown that caring for a child with a chronic condition such as eczema can actually have a positive influence on family functioning by uniting the family to interact more closely. What is crucial is having good-quality information about eczema, which your family can share to understand more about overcoming the condition. Having good knowledge about eczema in general has been shown to provide parents with a strong sense of control over the situation. Involve your other children as much as possible, and make sure their sleep is not being disturbed when their siblings' eczema flares up. Remember that there will be times when everything gets on top of you and relationships may temporarily run into difficulties, so ask your doctor or nurse for support during flare-ups if you feel things are getting out of control.

Q. My son loves having a bath with his older sister but always wants some of her bubble bath. I say no because I know it will irritate his skin, but this makes them fight. What can I do?

Try using an old bubble-bath container which has been washed out and rinsed well to put his bath oils/emollients in. If he sees that he will think he is having the same as his sister and they can both have a bath together. It is also fine for you to use the emollients to bathe your other children but remember to use a bath mat so they don't slip.

Q. Some of the treatments are very messy and greasy and I constantly have to battle with my son to put them on. This is causing so much stress between us – what can I do?

Many of the products used for children are very greasy. However, there is an enormous range of products available, from very light lotions to thick, ointment-based products (see treatment chapters). At the end of the day it is important you find one you both like, otherwise it will cause friction and resentment, and treatments will be left off. Ask your doctor or nurse if they have any samples you can try out. There is no reason why you can't have a selection of emollients so that the more acceptable ones can be used for daytime and the greasier ones for the night. Many doctors generally prefer to prescribe ointment-based steroids, but if you prefer a cream tell your doctor or nurse.

Q. My child is very clingy. Do you think this is because of his eczema?

Studies have shown that children with eczema are often more clingy and reliant on their mother. While this is sometimes related to a simple need for comfort, it may also be related to the way in which you interact with your child. Research has shown that many parents become overprotective of their children as a natural response to them having a medical condition. Parents may find it hard to let go in everyday situations, and don't give their children as much independence in daily activities such as washing and dressing. Although this protection is all done with the best intent in the world, it can encourage their children to become more dependent and reliant on them. Try to give your child some freedom and independence. This may include gradually encouraging him to take more control of his own skin, but it should also include activities unrelated to his eczema – perhaps going to a friend's house for tea or even a sleepover.

Q. My child always seems withdrawn and sad when he is with other children. He has had very severe eczema all his life and is on a restricted diet because of food allergies. How can I help him interact with other children?

There are a number of possible reasons for your child's behaviour, including low self-esteem, anxiety and even depression. It may help to invite one or two friends home to play to build up his confidence gradually as some children find big groups of friends intimidating. If he really does seem to want to be on his own all the time, discuss the problem with your doctor. Some children benefit from the input of a clinical psychologist to help uncover any underlying feelings or emotions that may be affecting their behaviour. Your GP or hospital doctor can arrange this if appropriate.

Q. My son's eczema is well controlled but I am sure he uses the scratching to manipulate me. Is there any help available?

Very occasionally children may scratch on purpose to get some positive gain from a situation, for example if they don't want to go somewhere, or want extra attention. It is always essential to ensure that their underlying eczema is perfectly controlled before you can attribute their scratching to manipulative behaviour. A combination of firm responses from you and positive feedback for not scratching is usually enough to discourage this behaviour. If the manipulation becomes a problem your doctor may recommend referral to a paediatric clinical psychologist who can spend time with you and your son, and talk through any underlying issues.

Q. My mother died recently and since then my eczema has been difficult to manage. Is my eczema flare-up likely to be related to her death?

Yes, this is very likely. Although stress is not a cause of eczema, any life events such as the loss of loved one, exams and illness do appear to make eczema worse. Many parents and patients know when their eczema will flare up and can often relate it to such major events. You may not feel motivated to care for your skin if other factors are playing a major part in your life but it is important you do or things will become out of control. Some people benefit from having someone regular to talk to about their loss (bereavement counselling); if you think this would be of help discuss this with your GP.

Q. I feel really fed up and depressed about how I look and feel. I know this is affecting my relationships with everyone around me. What can I do to help myself?

How we appear to others unfortunately influences their response to us and has a big impact on how we feel about ourselves. We live in an environment where body image and perfection are portrayed as important in many areas of everyday life such as advertising, magazines, films and TV. If you have a skin problem, the pressure of living up to this image of perfection is hard. You may not want to socialize or meet new people, and it is easy to find yourself avoiding relationships and shutting off from people. It is important you spend time with people who make you feel good about yourself and love you for who you are. By avoiding relationships you will make yourself feel even more insecure and create a vicious circle of low self-esteem. Don't bottle up your feelings – discuss them with your family, friends, nurse or doctor as they can all help in different ways. Finally, remember that there are many different treatment options available. Try to be positive about controlling your eczema, even if you feel totally fed up and can't be bothered to keep on top of your skin care. If you know your eczema isn't well controlled don't just assume that you've tried everything – speak to your doctor to discuss what other treatment options are available.

Summary

Eczema can have an impact on all areas of your life, and affects everyone in very different ways. Throughout the book the aim has been to help you understand your skin in a much deeper way and give you a comprehensive insight into every aspect of the condition, with practical advice on how to tailor treatment to your individual lifestyle. Overcoming eczema involves teamwork between healthcare professionals, family and friends, but remember that you are the most important person in this team and it is your knowledge and involvement that will make the biggest difference to your skin and your life.

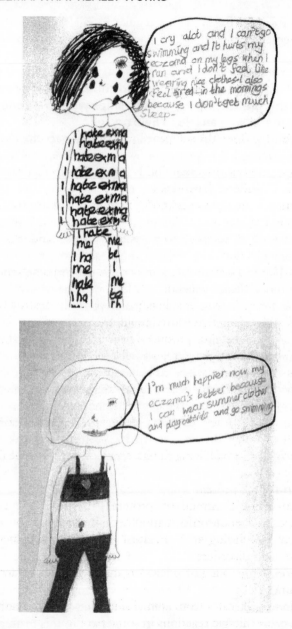

Overcoming eczema – the impact on a child's quality of life as seen through the eyes of Anna, aged 8

Glossary

Allergen (antigen) A substance (normally a protein) that causes an allergy

Allergy An abnormal reaction of the body to substances normally considered harmless

Anaemia A medical condition in which there are too few red cells in the blood

Anaphylaxis A serious and potentially life-threatening form of allergic reaction

Angioedema Deep swelling under the skin which can occur as part of an allergic reaction

Antibacterial A drug or substance designed to destroy bacteria

Antibiotic A drug that is used to kill bacteria and cure infections

Antibody A substance produced by the body to fight disease

Antihistamine A drug that is used to reduce inflammation caused by a chemical called histamine in the body

Antimicrobial A drug or substance used to destroy microscopic organisms such as bacteria, viruses and fungi

Atopic An inherited tendency to develop eczema, asthma or hayfever

Bacteria Very small living things, some of which cause illness or disease

Casein A milk protein

Chromosome A strand of protein found in body cells that carries the genetic information necessary for life

Clinical psychologist A therapist who deals with mental and emotional disorders

Culture The growing of micro-organisms such as bacteria in the laboratory

Dander Small scales from animal skins, hair or bird feathers that can cause allergic reactions in some people

Dermatitis Inflammation of the skin

Dermis The deep layer of the skin below the epidermis

Dietician A specialist in food and nutrition

Discoid Flat and circular or disc-shaped

Emollient An agent that softens or soothes the skin

Epidemiology The branch of medicine that deals with the study of the causes, distribution and control of disease in populations

Epidermis The outer layer of the skin

Exotoxin A toxic substance produced by micro-organisms

Fissure A break or split in the skin

Folliculitis Inflammation of the hair follicle

Gene A hereditary unit found on a chromosome that is responsible for passing on specific characteristics (such as hair colour) from parent to child

Generic drug A product which is not sold as a proprietary brand (trade name)

Genetics The study of how the qualities of living things are inherited or passed on through the genes

Herbalist Someone who grows, sells, or uses herbs, especially to treat illness

Histamine A chemical substance produced by the body during an allergic reaction

Hives A skin condition characterized by itchy skin lumps which can be caused by an allergic reaction (also called urticaria)

Homeopathy A system of medicine in which a disease is treated by giving extremely small amounts of a substance that causes the disease

Hyperpigmentation Increased skin pigmentation

Hypersensitivity An overreaction of the body to a normally harmless substance

Hypopigmentation Reduced skin colouration

IgE Immunoglobulin E, one of several types of antibody in the body

Immune Resistant to a particular disease owing to the body's production of antibodies or cells following previous exposure

Immunoglobulin A protein that is part of the immune system (also called an antibody)

Impetigo A bacterial skin infection caused by *Staphylococci* and *Streptococci* bacteria

Inflammation Red, painful, warm swelling of part of the body

Irritant A substance that can damage the skin surface

Lichenification Thickening of the skin caused by excessive scratching. The lines and markings of lichenified skin look more pronounced than usual

Lipid A fatty substance

Mast cells Cells found in the skin and airways which release histamine during an allergic reaction

Micro-organism A living thing that is so small that it cannot be seen without a microscope

Pompholyx A blistering eczema that affects the palms and soles

Pruritus Itching of the skin

Tachyphylaxis A decreasing response to a drug following administration of repeated doses

T-Cell A type of white blood cell called a lymphocyte that helps the body fight disease

Topical Applied to the skin surface

Toxin A poisonous substance produced by certain micro-organisms

Trade name (brand name) A proprietary name given to a particular product by the manufacturer

Urticaria A skin condition characterized by itchy skin lumps which can be caused by an allergic reaction (also called hives)

Wheal A small swelling on the skin that can be caused by an allergic reaction (also called welt)

Vesicle A small blister

Virus A very small micro-organism that causes infectious illnesses

Resources

National Eczema Society

The National Eczema Society is an organization in the UK dedicated to the needs of people with eczema and their carers. It provides practical information and support, along with booklets and fact sheets and runs a telephone helpline for patients and an information line for health professionals. Information on eczema and news updates can also be found on its website. The Society also provides an up-to-date list of companies manufacturing eczema products such as cotton clothing. In addition, the National Eczema Society funds research into the causes of eczema. The Society offers membership schemes for both patients and healthcare professionals.

National Eczema Society
Hill House
Highgate Hill
London N19 5NA
Telephone: 020-7281 3553
Eczema helpline: (0870) 241 3604 (Mon to Fri 8am to 8pm)
Fax: 020-7281 6395
Website: www.eczema.org
Email: helpline@eczema.org

Allergy UK

Allergy UK is a national medical charity established to increase understanding and awareness of allergy and to help people manage their allergies. The charity provides information on skin allergies, atopic eczema, anaphylaxis, and related atopic diseases such as asthma and hayfever.

Allergy UK
3 White Oak Square
London Road
Swanley
Kent BR8 7AG
Allergy helpline: (01322) 619898
Fax: (01322) 663 480
Website: www.allergyuk.org
E-mail: info@allergyuk.org

Anaphylaxis Campaign

The Anaphylaxis Campaign is an independent charity guided by leading UK allergists to support people who have life-threatening allergic reactions.

The Anaphylaxis Campaign
PO Box 275
Farnborough
GU14 6SX
Telephone: (01252) 373793
Helpline: (01252) 542029
Fax: (01252) 377140
Website: www.anaphylaxis.org.uk
Email: info@anaphylaxis.org.uk

Asthma UK

Asthma UK is a registered charity that can provide you with up-to-date information about asthma.

Asthma UK
Summit House
70 Wilson Street
London EC2A 2DB
Telephone: 020-7786 4900
Supporter & information team: 020-7786 5000
Advice line: (08457) 01 02 03
Fax: 020-7256 6075
Website: www.asthma.org.uk

BestTreatments

BestTreatments is a website linked to NHS Direct Online (see page 203). It is designed to help you and your doctor use high-quality evidence from medical research to decide together which treatments are best for you. The website contains excellent evidence-based information on the prevention and treatment of eczema. The information is based on *Clinical Evidence*, a publication produced by the British Medical Journal (BMJ) Publishing Group.

Website: www.besttreatments.co.uk

British Association of Dermatologists

The British Association of Dermatologists is a long-established association of practising UK dermatologists (skin specialists) which aims to continually improve the treatment and understanding of skin disease. The website provides a number of information sheets about eczema, written and approved by practising dermatologists, as well as general information about the skin, dermatology in the UK, and current issues in skin disease.

British Association of Dermatologists
4 Fitzroy Square
London W1T 5HQ
Telephone: 020-7383 0266
Fax: 020-7388 5263
Website: www.bad.org.uk
Email: admin@bad.org.uk

British Dermatological Nursing Group

The British Dermatological Nursing Group (BDNG) was established in 1989 to offer an independent speciality group for nurses and healthcare professionals with an interest in dermatology.

British Dermatological Nursing Group
4 Fitzroy Square
London W1T 5HQ
Telephone: 020-7391 6340
Website: www.bdng.org.uk
Email: admin@bad.org.uk

British Homeopathic Association

The British Homeopathic Association can provide a list of all homeopathic practitioners that are members of the Faculty of Homeopathy. All practitioners in the Faculty of Homeopathy are registered with a statutory professional body and have undertaken training in homeopathy at a Faculty-accredited postgraduate teaching centre.

British Homeopathic Association
Hahnemann House
29 Park Street West
Luton LU1 3BE
Telephone: (0870) 444 3950
Fax: (0870) 444 3960
Website: www.trusthomeopathy.org

Changing Faces

Changing Faces is a national charity based in the UK that provides support for people with disfiguring skin conditions, including eczema. The charity has pioneered a unique programme of disfigurement life-skills for children, young people, adults and families to support people in developing their self-confidence and self-esteem. This is offered through life skills workshops and regional days, counselling and self-help guides.

Changing Faces
The Squire Centre
33–37 University Street
London WC1E 6JN
Telephone: (0845) 4500 275
Fax: (0845) 4500 276
Website: www.changingfaces.org.uk
Email: info@changingfaces.org.uk

Department for Work and Pensions

The Department for Work and Pensions can provide up-to-date information on the range of benefits and services available for people who are sick or have a disability.

Attendance Allowance and Disability Living Allowance
Warbreck House
Warbreck Hill
Blackpool
Lancashire
FY2 0YE
Benefit Enquiry Line
Telephone: (0800) 882200
General enquiries about Attendance Allowance and Disability Living Allowance
Telephone: (08457) 12 34 56
Website: www.dwp.gov.uk

MHRA (Medicines & Healthcare products Regulatory Agency)

The MHRA is an executive agency of the Department of Health. It is responsible for protecting and promoting public health and patient safety by ensuring that medicines, healthcare products and medical equipment meet appropriate standards of safety, quality, performance and effectiveness, and are used safely. The MHRA provides excellent, up-to-date information on the safety and regulation of herbal medicines.

Information Centre
Medicines and Healthcare product Regulatory Agency
10–2, Market Towers
1 Nine Elms Lane
London SW8 5NQ
Telephone: 020-7084 2000
Fax: 020-7084 2353
Website: www.mhra.gov.uk
Email: info@mhra.gsi.gov.uk

The National Electronic Library for Health (NLH) Skin Disorders Specialist Library

The National Electronic Library for Health Skin Disorders Specialist Library is intended to be a one-stop resource for quality, evidence-based information on dermatology that is relevant to UK health professionals. The Skin Conditions Specialist

Library provides an organized, easily accessible and up-to-date collection of key documents, reviewed evidence and appraised information on skin conditions, including selected patient information resources.

Website: http://libraries.nelh.nhs.uk/skin/

NHS Direct
NHS Direct operates a 24-hour nurse advice and health information service. This provides information on a number of health conditions including eczema, and details of local healthcare services such as doctors, late-night-opening pharmacies and self-help organizations.

Telephone service: (0845) 4647
Website: www.nhsdirect.nhs.uk

National Institute for Health and Clinical Excellence (NICE)
NICE is an independent UK organization responsible for providing national guidance on the promotion of good health and the prevention and treatment of ill health. NICE guidance is developed using the expertise of the NHS including NHS staff, healthcare professionals, patients and carers, industry and the academic world. A number of guidelines relating to eczema are now available from NICE. These include guidance on the use of topical steroids and topical immunomodulators, and guidance on referral of patients with eczema from GP to hospital-based care.

NICE
MidCity Place
71 High Holborn
London WC1V 6NA
Telephone: 020-7067 5800
Fax: 020-7067 5801
Website: www.nice.org.uk
Email: nice@nice.nhs.uk

Skin Care Campaign

The Skin Campaign (SCC) is made up of patient groups and other organizations with an interest in skin diseases. It makes recommendations for improvements in dermatology services to the government, and runs media campaigns and Skin Information Days for health professionals and the public. It does not provide information or answer queries about individual skin diseases.

Skin Care Campaign
Hill House
Highgate Hill
London N19 5NA
Website: www.skincarecampaign.org

Society of Homeopaths

The Society of Homeopaths is the largest organization registering professional homeopaths in the UK, and can provide you with an up-to-date list of registered homeopaths near your home.

The Society of Homeopaths
11 Brookfield
Duncan Close
Moulton Park
Northampton NN3 6WL
Telephone: (0845) 450 6611
Fax: (0845) 450 6622
Website: www.homeopathy-soh.com
Email: info@homeopathy-soh.org

Systematic Review of Treatments for Atopic Eczema

This document is a comprehensive summary of all the high-quality research trials investigating treatments for atopic eczema up until the year 2000. The systematic review was produced in collaboration with the Department of Health, and is a useful source of information for both patients and healthcare professionals.
Website: www.ncchta.org/execsumm/summ437.htm

Index

aciclovir 51, 52, 117
acne 72, 93, 110, 175–6
acupuncture 126–7
adhesives 167
adrenaline 134, 135, 148, 163
after-shaves 174
age
    and asteatotic eczema 14
    and atopic eczema 6
    and seborrhoeic eczema 9
ageing, premature 108, 171
air conditioning 170
air travel 170, 172
alcohol, and topical immunomodulators
    93
allergic contact dermatitis 10–12, 151
    and choice of career 166–7
    and delayed allergy 136, 151
    and food additives 147
    and footwear 161
    and leg ulcers 11, 16
    and nickel 152, 174–5
    patch-testing for 10, 90, 138
allergy
    allergy tests 137–54
        blood tests for specific IgE 137,
            139, 140–2, 143
        by alternative practitioners 139–40
        interpreting results 141–2, 143
        patch-testing 10, 23–4, 90, 138,
            140, 142
        photopatch-testing 172
        side-effects 140
        skin-prick tests 137–8, 140–1
    definition 4, 132–4
    growing out of 146–7
    role of in eczema 134–6
    symptoms of 133, 135, 136

    to antibiotics 78
    to bandages 101
    to emollients 66, 67
    to food 4, 37–40, 129, 136, 142–9
    to house dust mites 23, 136, 150
    to pets 33–4, 151
    to topical steroids 73–4, 154
    see also delayed allergies; immediate
        allergies
Allergy UK 136, 198–9
alternative treatment and interventions
    118–31
    allergy testing 139–40
    complementary therapies 118–27
    dietary interventions 129–30
    psychological approaches 127–8
    salt baths 130–1
anaemia 114
anaphylaxis 134, 135, 140
Anaphylaxis Campaign 136, 199
angioedema 133
animals
    allergies to 33–4, 151
    careers involving 166
antibacterial agents
    in emollients 65–6
    in topical steroids 77–8
antibiotics
    intravenous 50
    oral 47, 78, 116
    resistance to 48–9
    in topical steroids 48, 73, 77–8
antibodies 6
antifungal agents, in topical steroids 78
antifungal tablets 117
antihistamines 35, 115–16, 140, 166
    for sleep problems 115, 179, 180
antioxidants 147

antiviral tablets 51, 52, 116–17
anxiety 184–6
applied kinesiology 139
aqueous cream 67
arachis oil 149
arnica 123
aromatherapy 125
art and crafts 157, 163
asteatotic eczema 14
  emollients for 69
  and washing 28, 30
asthma 4–5, 6, 8, 133, 142
  and house dust mites 22, 23
  and oral steroids 109
  and pets 34
  and pollution 37
Asthma UK 199
athlete's foot 17, 55, 161
atopic eczema 3–8
  allergy and 134–6
  common sites of 4
  diagnosis of 5–6
  dietary factors 37–40, 142
  duration of 8
  environmental factors 22, 22–37
  genetic factors 6–7, 20–1
  and hygiene hypothesis 40–2
  incidence of 3–5, 6–8
  and other atopic diseases 4–5
  and topical immunomodulators 95
atopic winter feet see juvenile plantar
      dermatosis
atopy patch test 24, 138
Attendance Allowance and Disability
      Living Allowance 202
azathioprine 114–15
  duration of use 115
  and other medicines 115
  side-effects 114–15

baby wipes 28
bacterial infections 46–50
  antibiotic-resistant 48–9
  and oral antibiotics 116
  prevention of 50
  recognizing 46
  transfer of 50
  treatment of 47–9
bandages 61, 68, 100–6, 162, 179
  compression bandages 105–6
  dry-wrap bandages 103–4
  medicated bandages 104–5
  use of topical immunomodulators
      under 96
  use of topical steroids under 96–7,
      101
  wet-wrap bandages 100–3
  when to use 101–2
baths
  frequency of 27, 187
  salt 130–1
  use of emollients in 64, 65
BCG vaccination 97
bedding 24–5, 36, 170, 180
bedrooms, temperature of 35–6, 170,
      179–80
behavioural modification techniques 60,
      127–8
benefits, disability 201–2
benzoic acid 147
bereavement 192–3
BestTreatments 200
Betnovate 84–5
bleaching agents 32
blinds 25
blood pressure, high 110, 112
blood sugar levels 110
blood tests 6
  on Chinese herbal medicines 123
  on immunosuppressants 112, 114
  for specific IgE 137, 139, 140–1, 143
body image 193
bone marrow 114
bones, thinning of 110
breastfeeding
  and development of allergies 39–40
  and probiotics 130
  and use of topical
      immunomodulators 97
  and use of topical steroids 97
British Association of Dermatologists
      200

British Dermatological Nursing Group 200
British Homeopathic Association 201
bubble bath 27–8, 65, 190–1
bullying 156
bunk beds 25

calcineurin inhibitors *see* immunomodulators, topical
cancer
    and immunosuppressants 112, 114–15
    see also skin cancer
candida 18, 55, 78
car mechanics 166
careers, choice of 166–7
carpets 24, 25
casein 147
cataracts 82
catering 166
cats 151
cavity-wall insulation 35
cement, and contact dermatitis 11, 167
central heating 35
Centre of Evidence-Based Dermatology 125
chamomile 123
Changing Faces 183, 201
chickenpox 52, 94, 110, 156–7
child development
    and topical immunomodulators 94
    and topical steroids 72, 185
children
    and allergy tests 140
    clingy 191
    growing up 173–7
    and immunosuppressants 113, 115
    and nursery and school 155–67
    and oral steroids 111
    and topical steroids 83–4, 86
Chinese herbal medicine 121–3
    safety of 122–3
    side-effects of 122
chlorine 168, 172
ciclosporin 52, 94, 111–14
    duration of use 113

and other medicines 113–14
    side-effects 112
cinnamon flavouring 147
cleaning products 30–1
Clinical Evidence 200
clinical psychologists 60, 192
clothing 33, 159, 169
coal tar preparations *see* tar preparations
cold sores 51–2, 94, 117
colourings, food 147
communication, breakdown of 189
complementary therapies 118–27
    acupuncture 126–7
    aromatherapy 125
    Chinese herbal medicine 121–3
    finding a good practitioner 119–20
    general advice on 127
    herbal medicines 123–4
    homeopathy 124–5
    hypnotherapy 126
    massage 125–6
    NHS availability of 119, 121, 124, 129
    reflexology 126
compression bandages/stockings 15, 43, 105–6
concentration problems 187
contact dermatitis 9–12
    avoidance of 12
    common causes of 11
    duration of 12
    emollients for 68–9
    incidence of 11
    types of 9–10
    see also allergic contact dermatitis; irritant contact dermatitis
contact urticaria 149, 157
corticosteroids *see* steroids, topical
cosmetics, allergy to 153, 175
cotton clothing 33, 159
covers, for bedding 24–5, 26
cradle-cap 8, 68
curtains 25

dandruff 16
Dead Sea 131

deep vein thrombosis, and gravitational
    eczema 15, 43, 106
delayed allergies 133–4, 136
    patch-testing for 138
Department for Work and Pensions
    201–2
depilatory hair-removal products
    174
depression 182–3, 193
dermatologists 58–9
    and patch-testing 139
    referral guidelines 59
dermatology nurse specialists 59–60
dermis 2
detergents 30–2
diabetes 110
diesel 37
dietary factors 37–40
dietary interventions 129–30
dieticians 60, 143, 144
dinners, school 163–4
discoid eczema 12–13
    common sites of 4
    duration of 13
    incidence of 12
    and topical steroids 90–1
dishwashers 69
Doppler test 105
double-glazing 35
dry-wrap bandages 103–4
dyshidrotic eczema see pompholyx
    eczema

ears, piercing 174–5
eczema
    appearance of 2
    causes and prevention of 20–44
        dietary factors 37–40
        environmental factors 22–37
        genetic factors 20–2
        gravity 42–3
        reduced exposure to infection
            40–2
        stress 43–4
    common sites of 4
    damage caused to skin by 2–3

definition of 1
and infections 45–55
no cure for 56, 74–5
other conditions mistaken for
    16–19
psychological aspects of 178–94
sources of information 198–204
treatment
    general advice 56–61
    general order of treatments 61
    written record of 78, 81
    see also alternative treatments and
        interventions; bandages;
        emollients; immunomodulators,
        topical; light therapy; steroids,
        topical; tablet treatment
types of 3–16
    see also asteatotic eczema; atopic
        eczema; contact dermatitis;
        discoid eczema; gravitational
        eczema; pompholyx eczema;
        seborrhoeic eczema
eczema craquelé see asteatotic eczema
eczema herpeticum 51–2, 94, 116–17
education 155–67
egg allergy 38, 142, 145–6
    and immunization 42, 146
Elidel 51, 92–9
emollients 62–9
    antibacterial agents in 65–6
    and application of topical
        immunomodulators 95
    at school 159–60
    for the bath 64
    choice of 63–4, 191
    for different types of eczema 67–9
    as first line of treatment 60–1
    how to use 64–6
    massaging with 126
    and overheating 36
    in prevention of bacterial infection
        50
    for shaving 174
    side-effects 66
    as soap substitute 28, 63, 65
emotional effects of eczema 178–93

engineering 166
enzymes 32, 144
epidermis 2, 3
epinephrine 134, 135, 148, 163
epoxy resins 167
erythromycin 47, 116
essential fatty acids 129
essential oils 125
ethnicity, and atopic eczema 7
Eumovate 74
evening primrose oil 129
exams, school 165–6
exclusion diets 38, 129, 142–3, 144,
        163
exhaustion, of eczema sufferers and
        their carers 178–81
exotoxins 46
eyes
    and pollen allergy 151
    topical immunomodulators around
        98
    topical steroids around 82–3

fabric conditioners 33
face
    shaving 174
    use of topical steroids on 82, 189
family life, strain of eczema on 189–91
family size, and atopic eczema 7, 41
feet
    juvenile plantar dermatosis 161
    and pompholyx eczema 13
    use of topical steroids on 83
fingernails see nails
fingertip units 75
fish allergy 38, 142
flavour enhancers 147
flucloxacillin 47, 116
folliculitis 65, 68, 72, 87, 93, 174
food additives 147
food allergy/intolerance
    exclusion diets 129, 142–3, 144,
        163
    growing out of 146–7
    role in eczema 4, 37–40, 136, 142–9,
        170

symptoms 135, 136, 144
    testing for 141
food preparation 69, 166
food supplements 164
football 169
fragrances, and contact dermatitis 11
friendships 173, 188, 192
fruit
    and contact urticaria 149, 157
    irritant effect on mouth 147–8
frustration 187
fungal infections 55
fur 4, 33–4, 166
fusidic acid 48

gas fumes 37
gender
    and incidence of atopic eczema 7
    and incidence of seborrhoeic eczema
        9
general practitioners 57
    relationship with 187–8
    with special interest in dermatology
        58
generic names, topical steroids 79–81
genetic factors
    and atopic eczema 6–7, 20–1
    gene technology 21
    and seborrhoeic eczema 9
glaucoma 82
glues 167
grapefruit juice, and ciclosporin 114
grass pollen 160
gravitational eczema 14–16, 42–3
    common sites of 4, 14, 15
    duration of 15
    incidence of 15
    use of compression bandages for
        105–6
gravity 42–3
growth
    and oral steroids 110, 111
    and topical immunomodulators
        94
    and topical steroids 72, 185
guilt, parental 182–3

habit reversal 127, 128, 184–5
hair
    analysis of 139
    dyes 176–7
    growth, and topical steroids 72
    loss 17, 18
    removal 173–4
hairdressing 153, 166
hands
    and choice of career 166–7
    and contact dermatitis 10, 11, 31, 36,
        153
    contact urticaria 149
    emollients for 68–9, 90
    and playgroup activities 157
    and pompholyx eczema 13, 36, 89
    use of topical steroids on 83, 89, 90
hayfever 4–5, 6, 8, 116, 140, 142
head lice 164
health visitors 57–8
heating systems 26, 35, 170
herbal creams 123
herbal medicines 123–4
    see also Chinese herbal medicine
herpes simplex 51–2
herpes viruses 50–2, 94, 116–17
hives see urticaria
holidays 170–3
homeopathy 124–5, 201, 204
hospitals
    dermatology departments 58, 59–60
    other specialists 58–9
house dust mites 4, 20, 22–6, 136, 150
    allergy tests 141
    and pets 34
humidity 35, 69, 172
hydrocortisone 70, 74, 83–4, 154
hydrolysed formula milk 39
hygiene hypothesis 40–2
hypnotherapy 126
hypoallergenic products 175

'id' reaction 17
IgE (immunoglobulin E) 6, 22–3, 34, 37,
        133, 134, 147
    blood test for 137, 139, 140–2, 143

immediate allergies 23, 38, 133–4, 136
immune system
    and allergic contact dermatitis 10
    and bacterial infection 46–7
    and Chinese herbal medicine 121
    effect of topical immunomodulators
        on 92, 94
    and hygiene hypothesis 40–1
    overreaction in atopic diseases 4, 92,
        132–4
immunizations 42, 45, 97, 146, 157–8
immunoglobulin E see IgE
immunologists 59
    and skin-prick testing 139
immunomodulators, topical 60–1, 91,
        92–9
    advantages over topical steroids 93
    duration of use 95
    how they work 92–3
    how to use 95–7
    and immunization 97
    not for use on infected skin 94,
        98–9
    in prevention of flare-ups 97
    side-effects 93–5
    use in different types of eczema
        98–9
immunosuppressants 52, 94, 111–15,
        157
impetigo 49
income, relation to atopic eczema 6–7
indigestion 110
infections
    bacterial 46–50
    and eczema 45–55
    fungal and yeast 55
    and immunosuppressants 110, 157
    primary 45
    reduced exposure to and incidence of
        eczema 40–2
    secondary 45
    viral 50–5, 157
information, sources of 186, 198–204
irritability 186–7
irritant contact dermatitis 9–10, 11, 12
isotretinoin 176

itch-scratch cycle
  bandages and 101
  ciclosporin and 113
  habit reversal and 128, 184–5
  light therapy and 109
  and sleep problems 179–81

jewellery, and contact dermatitis 11, 152
juvenile plantar dermatosis 161

kidney damage 112, 122, 123
kinesiology, applied 139

latex allergy 150
legs
  and gravitational eczema 14–16, 43,
      105–6
  shaving 173–4
  ulcers
    and allergic contact dermatitis 11,
        16
    and gravitational eczema 15–16,
        43, 106
leisure activities 168–77
lichenification
  and emollients 68
  and medicated bandages 104
  and tar preparations 91
  and topical immunomodulators 98
  and topical steroids 85–6
  and wet-wrap bandages 102
light therapy 61, 107–9
  side-effects 108–9
lipids, in skin 2–3, 62
lips, swelling of 135, 136, 148, 151
liver, inflammation of 114, 117, 123
Locoid 85

make-up 153, 175
malassezia furfur 29, 55, 88
manipulative behaviour 192
marriages, strain of eczema on 189
massage 125–6
mattresses 24
measles vaccine 97
Medic Alert® bracelets 148, 150

medicated bandages 104–5, 162
messy play 157, 163
MHRA (Medicines and Healthcare
        products Regulatory Agency)
        124, 202
milk
  cow's 38, 39, 142, 144–5
  hydrolysed formula 39, 145
  soya 40, 145
mineral supplements 129
mittens, cotton 179
MMR vaccine 146
moisturizers *see* emollients
molluscum contagiosum 53–5, 94
mood changes 110
mould 37
mouth, soreness around 147–8
MRSA 49
mupirocin 48–9
mycobacterial vaccae injections 42

nails
  keeping short and clean 179, 184
  thickening 10, 16
nappies 158
nappy rash 18
National Eczema Society 121, 155, 159,
        183, 186, 198
National Electronic Library for Health
        (NLH) 202–3
National Institute for Health and
        Clinical Excellence (NICE) 204
NHS Direct 203
nickel 11, 151–2, 174–5
  in the diet 151–2
  problems of avoiding 151
nitrous oxides 37
nummular eczema *see* discoid eczema
nursery school 155–8
nursing (as a career) 166
nuts (tree) 38, 142, 148

occupational-related skin disease 11, 90,
        153, 166–7
oral allergy syndrome 151
organ transplants 111, 114

paediatricians 58
pancreas, inflammation of 114
parabens 147
parasite infections 41
paste bandages 91, 104–5
patch tests 10, 24, 90, 138, 140, 142
    photopatch-testing 172
    substances tested for 141
PE 160
peanut allergy 38, 39, 142, 148–9
    and arachis oil 149
penicillin 47
perioral dermatitis 72
pets 33–5, 151
pharmacists 60, 74
photopatch-testing 172
photosensitivity 108
phototherapy *see* light therapy
phytoestrogens 145
pigmentation, skin 72–3, 91
pillows 24
pimecrolimus *see* Elidel
plants, and contact dermatitis 11
plastering 167
playgroups 155–8
polio vaccine (oral) 97
pollen 4, 37, 136, 141, 151, 160
pollution 37
pompholyx eczema 13–14, 36
    and allergy 136
    duration of 14
    incidence of 13
    use of emollients in 89
    use of topical steroids in 89
post-inflammatory hyperpigmentation
        73, 91
post-inflammatory hypopigmentation
        73
potassium permanganate 89, 104–5
potty-training 158
pox virus 53
practice nurses 57–8
prednisolone 109, 111
pregnancy
    and Chinese herbal medicine 122
    and ciclosporin 112
    and development of allergies 38–9
    and house dust mites 26
    and maternal guilt 182
    and probiotics 130
    and use of topical
            immunomodulators 97
    and use of topical steroids 97
preservatives
    and contact dermatitis 11
    in emollients 66, 67
    in topical steroids 73, 76, 154
    and urticaria 147
probiotics 42, 130
protein contact dermatitis 149
Protopic 51, 92–9, 176
psoralen 108
psoriasis 16–17, 70, 91, 107
psychological impact of eczema
        178–94
psychological therapies 127–8
PUVA 108
pyridoxine 129

Qi 127
quality of life 178–94

race, and atopic eczema 7
reflexology 126
relationships 187–93
rings 69
ringworm 17–18, 55
Royal College of Nursing 119
rubber
    and allergic contact dermatitis 11,
        141, 150
    and contact urticaria 150
    gloves 31, 69, 150
rubella vaccine 97

saliva, animal 33–4
salt baths 130–1
scabies 18–19
scalded skin syndrome 49
scalp 8–9, 17–18, 29
    and hair dye 176–7
    and topical steroids 86–7

school 155–6, 159–67
  dinners 163–4
  exams 165–6
  problem activities 163
  trips 165
  uniform 159
sea water 131, 172
seborrhoeic eczema 8–9
  in adults 9
  and antifungal tablets 117
  in children 8–9, 88–9
  combined steroid/antifungal
      preparations for 78, 88–9
  common sites of 4, 8
  and shampoo 29
  and topical immunomodulators 99
selenium 129
self-esteem, low 192, 193, 201
shampoo 29
  tar-based 29, 68
shaving
  face 174
  legs 173–4
shellfish allergy 142
shin pads 169–70
shingles 94, 110
shoes, choice of 161
shower gels 27–8, 65
showers
  frequency of 27
  use of emollients in 64, 65
sibling rivalry 190
skin
  cross section of 1
  dry 14
  healthy 3
  infected 45–55, 94, 98, 102–3,
      161–2
  use of medicated bandages on
      104
  use of topical immunomodulators
      on 98–9
  use of topical steroids on 76–7
  use of wet-wrap bandages on 102
  thinning of see skin atrophy
skin atrophy 71, 101, 185

skin cancer
  and immunosuppressants 112, 114,
      115
  and light therapy 108, 109
  and topical immunomodulators 94
Skin Care Campaign 119, 204
skin creases
  and atopic eczema 5, 16
  and scalded skin syndrome 49
  and topical steroids 82
skin pigment, and topical steroids 72–3,
      91
skin-prick tests 137–8, 140–1
sleep
  and antihistamines 115–16
  problems with 178–81
sleepovers 173
soap 27–8, 65
social life 168–77
Society of Homeopaths 204
sodium benzoate 147
solid foods, introduction of 40
solvents 28
sorbic acid 147
soya allergy 38, 142, 145
sport 160, 161, 168–70
Staphylococcus aureus 46, 47, 49, 50
stasis eczema see gravitational eczema
steroids
  oral 52, 109–11
    precautions whilst taking 110–11,
      157
    side effects 109–10
  topical 70–91
    allergies to 73–4
    alternatives to 91
    and bandages 101
    basic rules for using 91
    and ciclosporin 113
    and duration of eczema 74
    duration of use 75
    how they work 71
    how to use 75–8
    and infected eczema 47–8
    non-prescription 74
    ointments versus creams 76, 191

steroids (*cont.*)
  topical (*cont.*)
    in preventative treatment 77
    recording treatment plan 78, 81
    reduced effectiveness over time 71
    side-effects 70, 71–3, 82, 185–6
    strengths of 70–1, 78–91
    table of combination 80–1
    table of plain 79–80
    use in adults 83–4
    use in babies 83
    use in children 83–4, 86
    value in treatment of eczema 60–1, 70, 74–5
stomach ulcers 110
Streptococcus 46, 47
stress 43–4, 125, 126, 165, 186–7, 192
stretch marks 71, 110, 185
striae *see* stretch marks
sulphites 147
sulphur dioxide 37
suncream
  allergy to 171–2
  choice of 171
  and topical immunomodulators 96
sunlight
  and contact dermatitis 12
  and improved eczema 37, 107, 171
  and skin cancer 95, 171
support stockings 15, 43, 105
surfactants 28, 32, 33
sweaty sock dermatitis *see* juvenile plantar dermatosis
swimming 168, 172
Systematic Review of Treatments for Atopic Eczema 204

T-cells (T-helper lymphocytes) 40–1, 46–7, 92, 112, 114, 133, 134
tablet treatment 109–17
  see also antibiotics, oral; antifungal tablets; antihistamines; antiviral tablets; immunosuppressants; steroids, oral
tachyphylaxis 71

tacrolimus *see* Protopic
tar preparations 29, 68, 91
tea tree oil 123
teasing 156, 162, 164
teenagers 165, 173–7
teething 158
telangiestasia 71, 82
temperature 35–6, 69, 162–3, 170, 179–80
  sensitivity to 93
textiles 33
thrush 18, 55, 78
thumb sucking 156
tiredness, of eczema sufferers and their carers 178–81
tobacco smoke 37
toenails, and fungal infections 55
topical therapies 60–1
  see also emollients; immunomodulators, topical; steroids, topical
toys, and house dust mites 25
travel insurance 170
treatments, eczema *see* alternative treatments and interventions; bandages; emollients; immunomodulators; immunosuppressants; light therapy; steroids; tablet treatment
tubular cotton bandages 100
tubular cotton garments 100

UK Atopic Dermatitis Diagnostic Criteria Working Party 5
ultraviolet light 107–9
uniform, school 159
urticaria 23, 34, 35, 38, 116, 133, 142, 145–6
  contact 147–8, 149, 157
UVA 107–8
UVB 107–8

vaccination *see* immunization
vacuuming 24, 25
varicose eczema *see* gravitational eczema

varicose veins, and gravitational eczema
15, 30, 43, 106
VEGA (or electrodermal) testing
139–40
vegetables, and contact urticaria 149,
157
ventilation 25, 180
vinyl flooring 24, 25
viral infections 50–5
vitamin E 129
vitamin supplements 129

wart viruses 53–5
washing
of bedding 25
of clothes 32, 33
see also baths; showers
washing machines 32–3

washing powder 31–3
water, in skin 2–3, 28
water quality 26–7
water softeners 27
waxing 174
weight gain, and oral steroids 110
wet-wrap bandaging 100–3, 162
how they work 100–1
side-effects 101
when to use 101–2
wheat allergy 38, 142
winter eczema *see* asteatotic eczema
worry 184–6

yeasts 8, 18, 29, 88, 89
and infections 55, 78

zinc 129